Dr. Vinod Verma

The Timeless Wisdom of Ayurveda
(A Scientific Exposition)

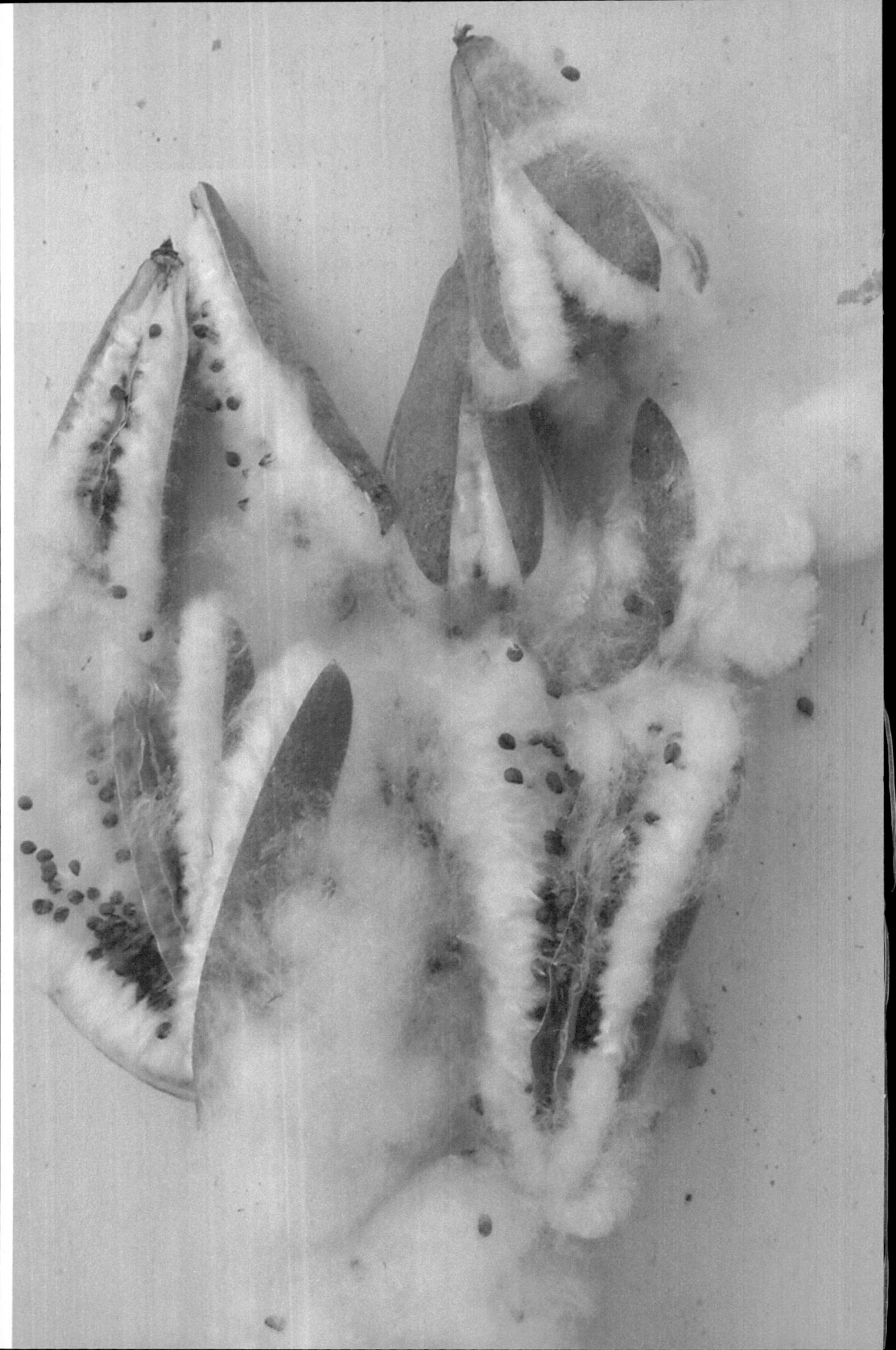

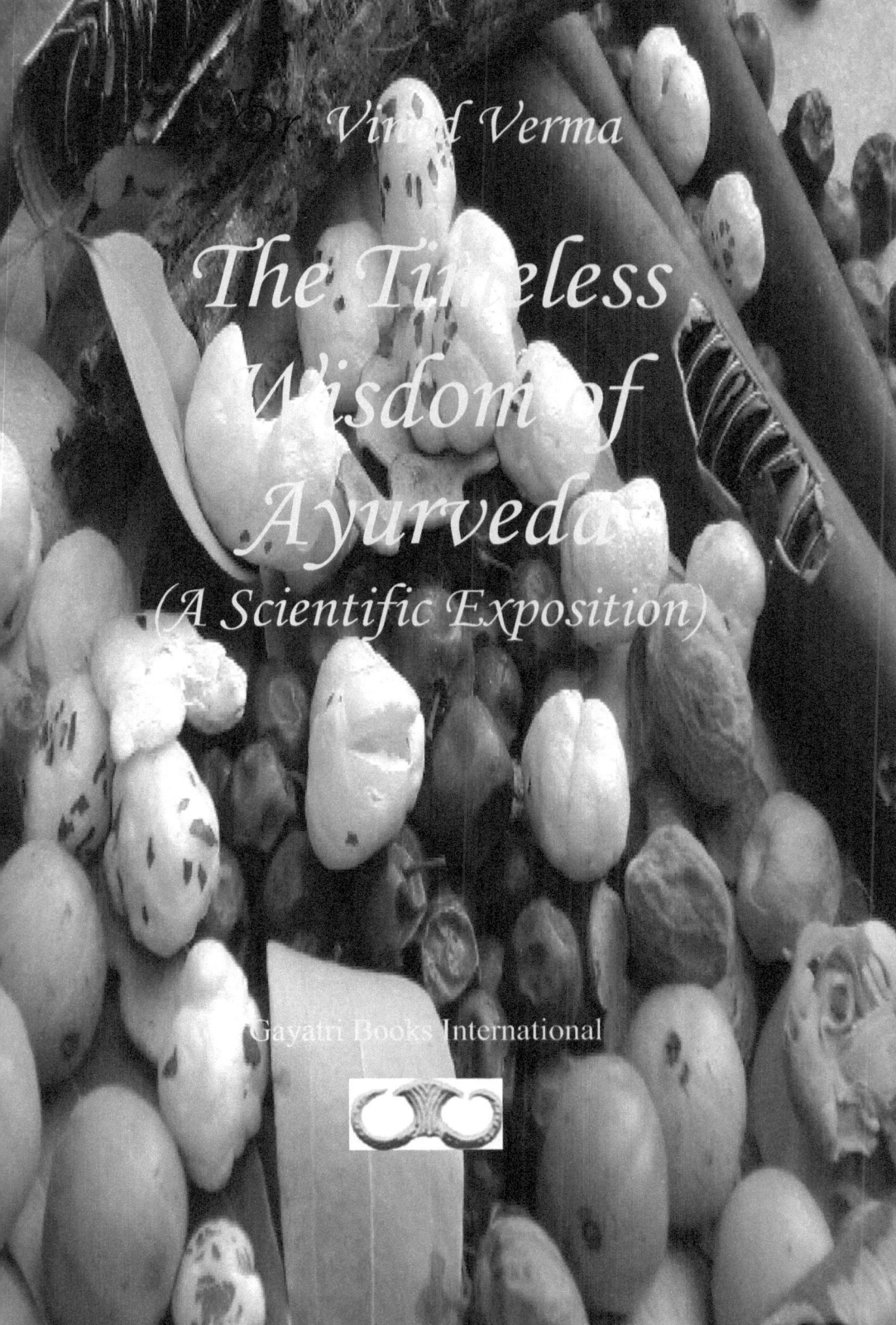

Dr. Vinod Verma

The Timeless Wisdom of Ayurveda

(A Scientific Exposition)

Gayatri Books International

The book is written for the purpose of education and self-help and not meant to replace the services of a physician. The author and the publisher are in no way responsible for any medical claims regarding the material presented in this book. For using methods provided in this book at commercial level requires the prior permission from the author. For more information, write to the author directly.

Visit Dr. Vinod Verma at www.ayurvedavv.com to find out about her other publications, seminars, lectures and consultations. Look for more information on the last pages of the book.

Translation rights are held by the author. Write to her at ayurvedavv@yahoo.com or ayurvedav@gmail.com.

Consultant: Mohit Joshi
Cover design and photographs by the author

ISBN: 9781494950668

Preface

Inspiration to write this book came several years ago after doing a daylong seminar in Dresden on 4th September 2004 for the Chamber of Pharmacists of Saxony as a part of their training programme. Some of my students, who have been studying Ayurveda with me for the last three years, told me that this form of condensed teaching had given them a lucid overview of the endless wisdom of Ayurveda. They suggested that a small booklet should be written to give an overview so that people can have a correct and scientific view of Ayurveda.

I wrote my first two books on Ayurveda in the late eighties and they were published also in different European languages in the early nineties, I was doubtful about the success of my labour abroad. On the contrary, these books became classics of Ayurveda for modern people, and led to the popularity of this ancient science of health and healing. However, after something becomes too popular, its depth and quality is lost and a superficial view predominates. Its sudden popularity during recent years in the West through Indian Gurus, Hotels and Women's magazines has given many misconceptions about Ayurveda. Wrongly, it is associated with religion, or merely massage or beauty or luxuries of maharajas, and so on. People, who want to have a lucid view of Ayurveda, sometimes find the big books formidable because of lack of time. Besides that, the market is flooded with non-scholarly books which provide further wrong notions about this scientific wisdom about health and healing from ancient India. I feel that this small book would be ideal for an empirical understanding of Ayurveda and would instigate people's awareness about their health and well-being, both home and abroad. The modern Indian folks or most metro dwellers are equally ignorant about the scientific wisdom of Ayurveda and the villagers of the post-independent India were fed on the colonial ideology that all indigenous wisdom is non-scientific and has lesser value.

This short and simple book can help people all over the world to comprehend the scientific and rational basis of Ayurveda and can help to integrate its simple practices in day-to-day life. It can initiate you to understand your first responsibility in life, which is towards your body. It is called svadharma (human duty for oneself) in Sanskrit. According to Ayurveda, **the first priority of life is life itself,** as when life is endangered with illness or it ends, the phenomenal world comes to an end for that particular person. It is our first duty to take care of our body and keep our thought process in equilibrium for maintaining health, enhance strength and live a long and peaceful life the optimum energy level.

I propose here a three-step process:
- attaining knowledge of the fundamentals of Ayurveda,
- understanding it from a cosmic prospective and not from the prospective of modern science which has a fragmented approach, and
- adopt some simple health practices to see the results for yourself.

You will find that some simple practices can make you feel better and can bring some change in your thinking. Ayurvedic wisdom would give you a better understanding of other human beings and that will help you to bring harmony and peace in your family life, as well as at your workplace and social surroundings. Thus, this book will help you understand that Ayurveda is not only a system of medicine from ancient India but it deals with every aspect of life. It is a system that deals with wisdom about the cosmos, life, health and healing. Mass education of Ayurveda will initiate people to take responsibility for their primary health into their own hands and use all means of preventive Ayurvedic practices to safeguard themselves from ailments and disorders. The aim of this book is to fill the gulf between body and mind and get rid of the attitude of comparing body to a machine and depending entirely on the medical community for its 'care and repair'.

Vinod Verma
July 2007
Ayurvedavv@yahoo.com
www.ayurvedavv.com
www.drvinodverma.com

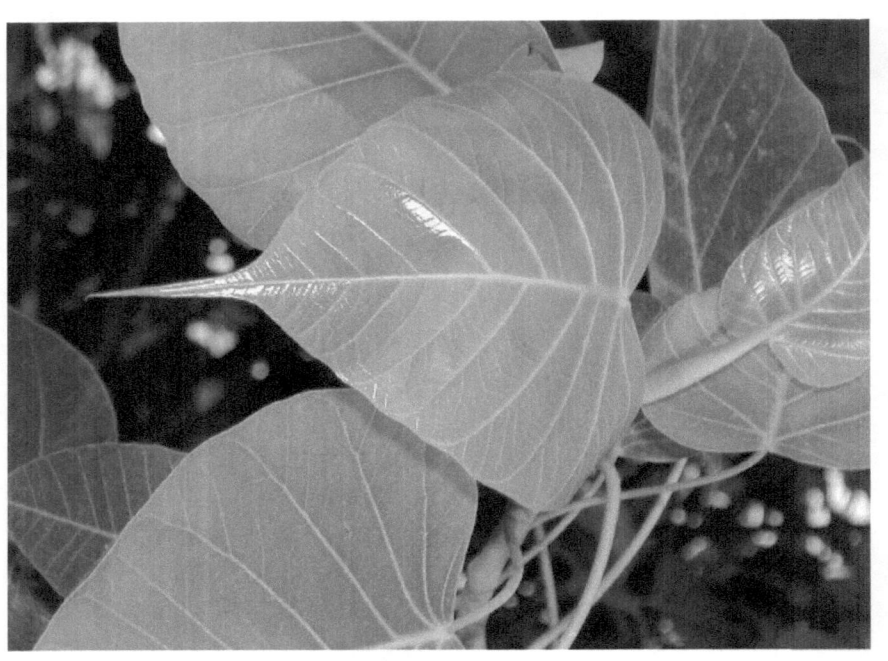

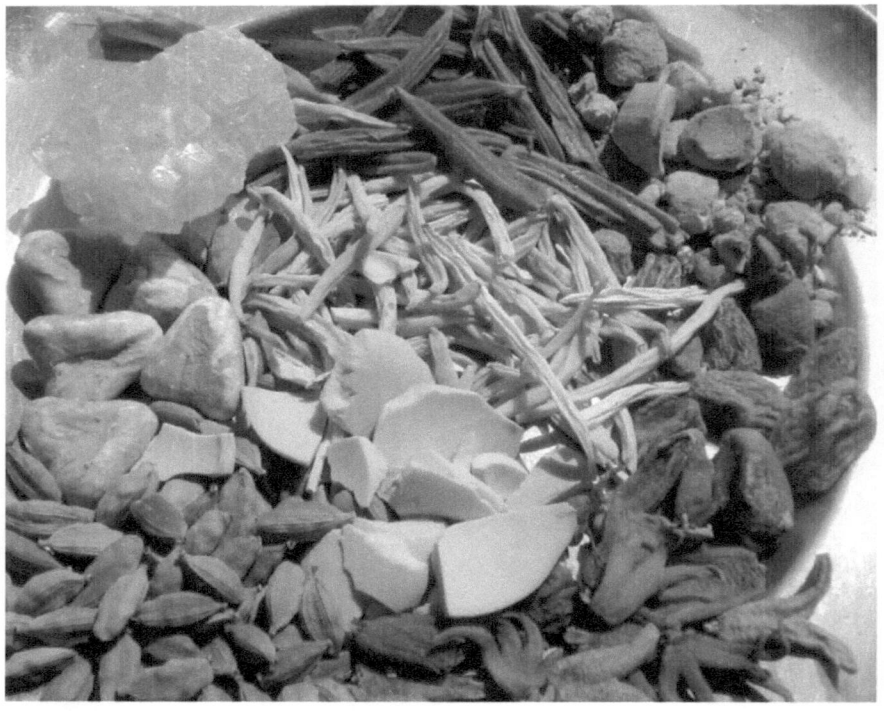

Contents

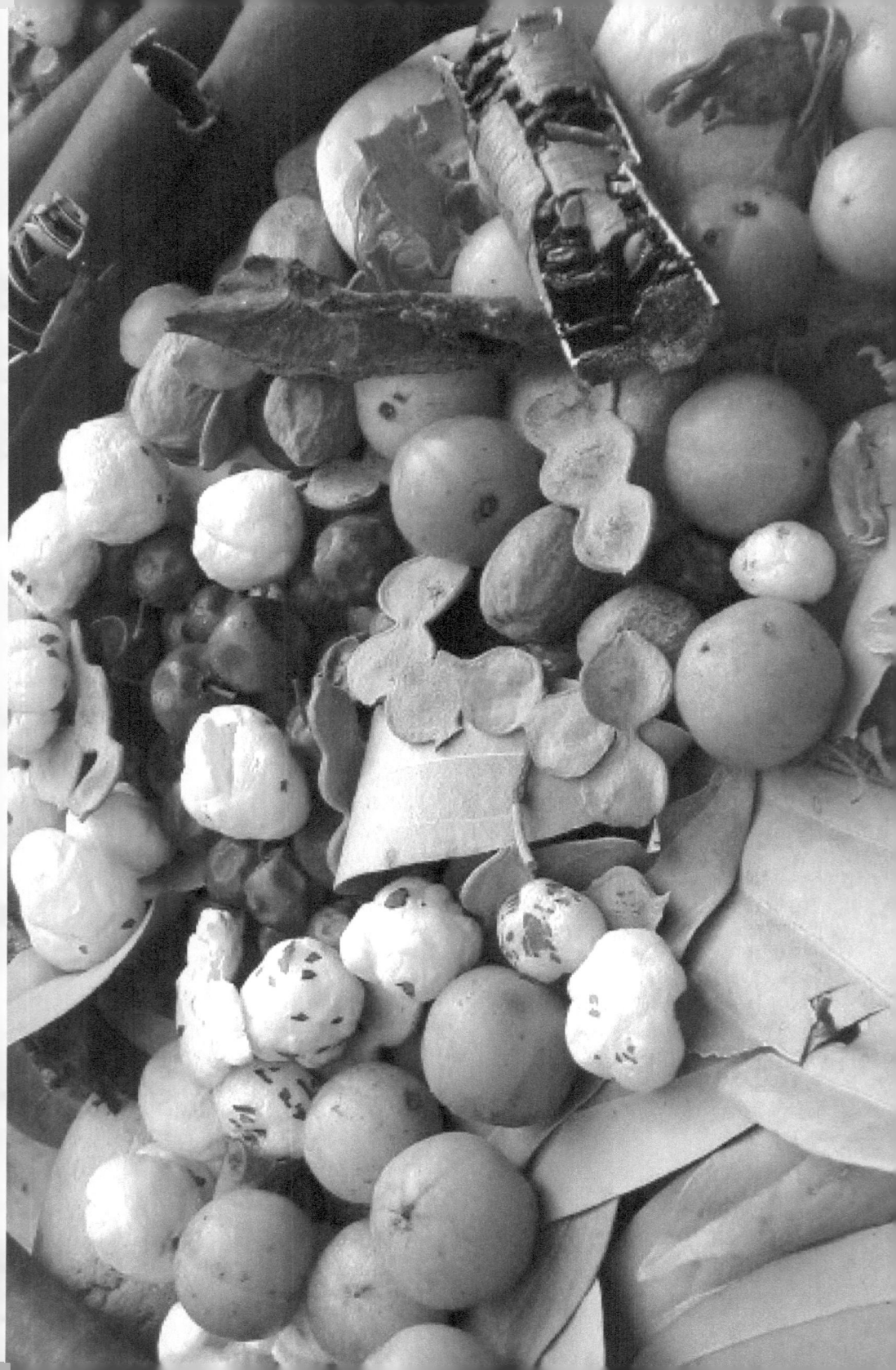

1
Ayurveda, the Universal Wealth from Ancient India

An individual's life span is the limited time period between birth and death. It is also called AAYU in Sanskrit. Veda means wisdom. Veda denotes both knowledge and science (*gyan* and *vigyan*). This should make clear the literal meaning of Ayurveda.

Ayurvedic concepts are based upon the fact that a single principal governs the whole cosmos and we are all interconnected, interrelated and inter-dependent. Well being of one is the well being of other existing thing and discomfort or disturbance is transferred to the others as well. We human beings along with other existing things in the cosmos are like glass balls in a jar with a narrow neck. It is difficult to take out one ball without disturbing the others. We are not superior to animals and plants. We are a tiny part of this infinite cosmos like anything else, as all that exists mutually affects, influences and interacts with each other. In many cultures of the world, human superiority over the rest is emphasized. Mahatma Gandhi said in beautiful words:

It is an arrogant assumption that human beings are lords and masters of the lower creatures... they are the trustees of the lower animal kingdom.

Many people around the world think that Ayurveda is a medical system from ancient India. In France, they always use the prefix medicine with Ayurveda (médicine ayurvedique). Ayurveda is not exclusively a system of medicine. It is the SCIENCE OF LIFE. It teaches you everything that belongs to life. I generally call it *a system of health and healing.* However, even this explanation is limited, as Ayurvedic wisdom from the scriptures also provides advice about the social aspects of life. You will find wisdom on environment and also about other aspects of the cosmos that affect life. Thus, Ayurveda has a broader spectrum than just dealing with ailments.

When we talk of the medical aspects of Ayurveda, the foremost emphasis is on maintaining health; what we call these days—the preventive medicine. In fact, most of the minor ailments are due to small imbalances in the body. These imbalances are generally created due to our negligence. To maintain the natural balance of the body, Ayurveda prescribes two principal things: Aahar and Vyavahar (Nutrition and lifestyle). It is not the lifestyle in its literal meaning, but much more than that, as it involves also your behaviour and thinking process. In Ayurveda, many diverse aspects are dealt with in detail—how do you wake up, what are your thoughts, what do you do after waking up, how do you breathe, how do you eat, what do you eat, where do you eat, how much do you eat, how do you deal with your work, your posture while working, how do you create a balance between your life at work and life at home, how do you manage stress, how do you walk and how do you talk, how do you prepare yourself to go from waking up mode to the sleep mode and many more aspects of life are dealt with.

The cosmos is dynamic and it has a rhythm. With all the actions and activities, it is like a big orchestra. We have to be in tune with the cosmic rhythm and if we are not in rhythm with the rest, we get out of tune. We are no more in harmony with the rest of the system. This is a state of being unwell. If an individual stays out of rhythm for a long time, he or she develops an ailment or a disorder. A smaller, independent sub-system develops in the body which is expressed in the form of pathology.

Treatment of ailments has an entirely different approach in Ayurveda. The person is treated and not exclusively the ailment. An ailment is a part of a person and is not viewed as independent. Along with the ailment, one has to take into consideration the rest of a person's body, mind, past and present social surroundings, and so on.

Let me give you a living example from the practice of an Ayurvedic physician called *Vaidya*. A person goes to a Vaidya and complains that he has headache. The vaidya who has already had a good look at the person and gathered enough information, feels the pulse and tells him—*your liver is not functioning properly*. The patient repeats—*I have headache and I am unable to work properly due to that*. The Vaidya says—*you also suffer from constipation and partial evacuation*. If a patient is not used to the holistic science of Ayurveda, he may feel irritated and may be willing to leave the place by then. Normally a good Vaidya explains by then, how the internal atmosphere of the body is polluted due to the malfunction of *agni* (the digestive fire of the body) and becomes the cause of a headache. In this particular case, the body is cleaned with a mild purgative, diet is changed and some medication is given to enhance the agni. The patient not only gets rid of his headache but also acquires a better complexion and appearance with this treatment.

Let us take a similar example in the allopathic treatment, which is not holistic but is based upon the treatment of symptoms. The person with a headache is given painkillers. If the patient returns to the doctor after two weeks and says that his headache is better when he takes the tablets, otherwise it returns, the patient is asked to do certain tests and is also given vitamin-mineral supplements along with the painkillers. If the headache still persists, the patient is sent for a CAT scan and other advanced tests. If nothing is found through all these expensive and time consuming tests, the source of ailment is said to be mental and generally the patient is recommended to psychiatry. In other words, when nothing is found at the finest level with all the tests, it is presumed that the patient has mental problems. A German psychiatrist colleague once rightly put it by saying that psychiatry is dustbin of the society.

It is often observed that due to a fragmented approach to allopathic treatment in our times, minor and simple to cure disorders are exaggerated and through all the tests an average patient is directed to undertake, he or she goes through a considerable amount of fear and tension.

I sum up below the importance of Ayurveda:
Ayurveda is the wisdom about life from ancient India. Whatever the geographical origin, the wisdom from the ancient world is our universal heritage. Ayurveda tells us the art, as well as the craft of living. When there arise hindrances like mental or physical pain, disorders, ailments and diseases; it provides remedies for them and prescribes methods

to bring the body to equilibrium and harmony again. Ayurveda also includes the science of rejuvenation in order to enhance vitality and minimise the effects of ageing. Ayurveda is a comprehensive science of life that also provides suggestions about how to live an enriched, happy and disease-free life and how to enhance the pleasures of life. It also instructs on optimising the quality of life and enhancing one's life span. All this is not only done with remedies of natural origin and balanced nutrition but also with one's mental and spiritual efforts. The scriptural wisdom of Ayurveda deals with the totality of life relating to physical and mental health, family structure, social situations, environment, and spiritual development.

Ayurveda in Europe

Exchange of Medical wisdom between Europe and India is very ancient. At the time of Hippocrates (460 to 377 BC), there was a regular exchange between Ayurvedic and Greek sages of medicine. It is known that Hippocrates travelled widely to Asia and had a holistic approach to medicine, which had parallels with Ayurveda. As in Ayurveda, Hippocrates had also described in his famous aphorisms the different human constitutions. This time was the golden period of Ayurveda. In addition to that, the Ayurvedic classical literature was translated into Arabic, which influenced the Arabic, as well as the Greek medicine*. In turn, Ayurveda was enriched with the wisdom of medicinal plants from Europe and the Middle East. There are many instances where medical wisdom related to these plants was

---

* *History of Medicine in India*, Editor, P.V. Sharma, 1992, Indian National Science Academy, New Delhi.

lost in their home countries but it was preserved and enriched by Ayurvedic sages.

Scientific valediction of Ayurveda

Many people in the world confuse Ayurveda with herbal medicine or other similar methods of healing. Herbal medicine or the many other healing methods from folklore traditions of the world are prescriptions of certain plant medicines for ailments or are description of methods or ceremonies for healing. They are not complete scientific systems like Ayurveda where aetiology of diseases, pharmacology of the medicinal substances, doses, toxicology, nutrition in relation to time, place and special circumstances, surgery, psychology, psychiatry, social behaviour and responsibilities of physicians, as well as of patients and hundreds of other related themes are described. In Ayurveda, it is advised that rational, mental and spiritual therapies should be applied simultaneously and not independently of each other. I cite below the views of Acharya Priya Vrat Sharma on the holistic and scientific approach of Charaka Samhita:

'The law of uniformity of nature was established which helped in applying the physical laws to the biological field. It remains a mystery for all in what type of laboratories and with what equipment they were able to arrive at these scientific truths. Perhaps the entire nature was their laboratory and their own keen observations and divine vision worked as their instruments.

...In order to stabilise the idea (of rationality), 'yukti' was added to one of the pramanas (means of valid knowledge). Caraka has emphasised all through to work according to yukti (rationale).

He has advised (us) to move always with knowledge. There should be a proper correlation of theoretical knowledge (jnana) and practical skill. Caraka has emphasised on the process of investigation which is essential for arriving at scientific truths...'

Many people think that Ayurveda propagates ahimsa (non-violence) and suggests following a vegetarian diet or is associated with some religion, and so on. These are absolutely false notions, and reasons for these are that many times Ayurveda is brought to the West through religious gurus and it is tinged with sects or religions and with their own specific interpretations. Charaka Samhita has the description of all kinds of meats and wines*. Ayurveda emphasises on the sensuous joy and besides foods and wines, there are parts on rejuvenation and sexuality. Ayurveda is about nature and the natural ways of building strength, enhancing sensuous joy, healing and treatment. Study of Charaka Samhita reveals that it does not have any moral, religious or philosophical biases. However, compared to the western scientific wisdom, Ayurveda has different fundamental principles and these are based upon the uniformity of the cosmos and the cosmos being a dynamic whole.

Holistic view of life

Modern medicine is based upon the concept that the cosmic reality is material and that it can be approached with senses. The material reality can be split into further fragments up to atoms and so on. Both, the cosmos and the human body work like a

---

* For more details, see my books: *Ayurveda: A Way of Life* and *Ayurveda for Inner Harmony*.

machine and time is conceived as linear. Ailments and disorders are recognised with their objective and measurable symptoms and thus treatment is given on the basis of these symptoms. Discomfort or illness is seen as the mal-functioning of the body-machine. Different mechanisms of the body are understood at biological and molecular levels and disorders are treated with physical or chemical intervention. Both, time and matter are reduced to smaller units and chance plays an important role in causing malfunctions and disorders.

Contrary to the above views, in the holistic system of Ayurveda, an individual is considered as a non-divisible unity, an integral whole which cannot be reduced in terms of its parts, nor can the individual be separated from the social, cultural and spiritual environment and the cosmic link. An illness is viewed as the consequence of disharmony with the cosmic order. It does not occur by chance and it is not limited to space and time. Matter is inter-linked, interconnected, interdependent and dynamic and it is this transformation that denotes time. Time is not linear but cyclic. For understanding malfunctions and for their treatment, the social, cultural and spiritual environments of an individual are taken into consideration.

2
Principle of Oneness in Dynamic Cosmos

In the cosmos, everything is interconnected and interdependent and works on the same principles. There is a cosmic unity in structure and function of all what exists. Thus, the principles that govern the cosmos also govern the human body. In a big cosmic system, our body is a smaller but independent cosmic system. The bigger and the smaller are all interconnected, interrelated and interdependent. The causative factor of the basic cosmic unity is the common constituent of all that exists.

The five elements or mahabhutas constitute the material reality of the universe. These are ether (space), air, fire, water and earth. Without space nothing can exist. It is the primary factor. In space there is air. Fire needs both air and space to exist. The fourth element, water, is dependent on its existence on the previous three elements. Water has also the warm element. Think of the ice age and how everything came to existence after that. The earth is the fifth element and heaviest of all. It needs all the other four elements for its existence and is comprehensive.

Five elements in the cosmos are dynamic and well coordinated and form a perfected system. The sun brings us warmth and light each day and the darkness of the night is beautified with stars and the changing phases of the moon. There are clouds, rain, snow and the rivers are gushing towards their destination. From the dynamism of the five elements, seeds become sprouts; trees lose their leaves and get new ones. The living being from both plant and animal worlds die and new life comes to being. There is no still moment in this dynamic cosmos and change is another name for time. Nothing is lost and there is constant transformation.

The Living systems with five Cosmic Elements

Like the cosmos, an individual living system is also perfect and dynamic. It is a part of the cosmos and likewise it is constituted of the five fundamental elements. But the elements in a living system are present in the form of three vital forces or energies called *doshas* in order to perform all the functions of this particular system.

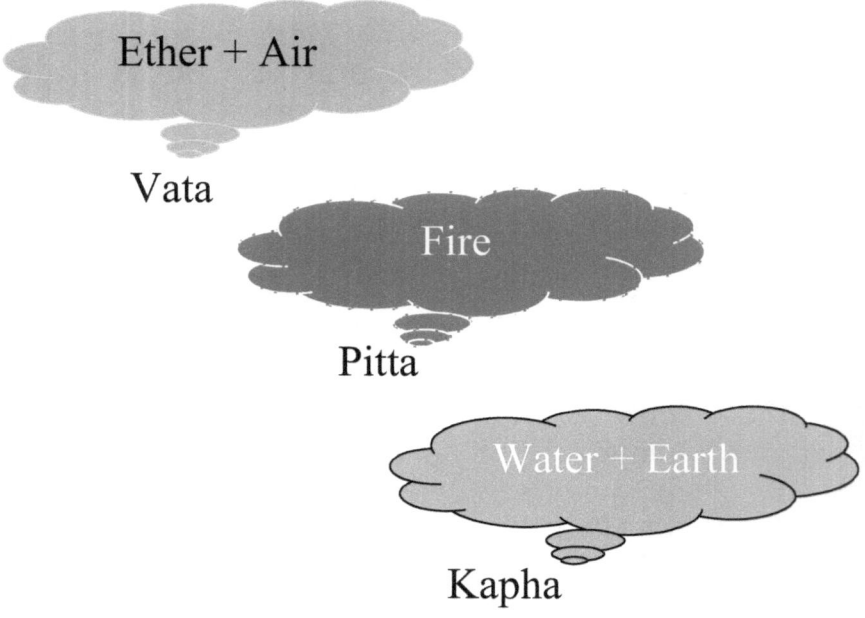

To perform all the mental and physical functions of the body, the three energies coordinate with each other and make a perfect system. The body has further smaller systems or organisms, which perform their individual functions, and the three vital forces also coordinate these functions. These energies are called **vata**, **pitta** and **kapha** and each has functions like the characteristics of the elements they are derived from.

Functions of vata, pitta and kapha

Vata is constituted from the elements ether and air and its functions are related to these two elements. Ether or space is omnipresent and air is mobile. The functions related to movements as well as to space are performed by vata.

> **Vata** is responsible for all body movements, blood circulation, respiration, excretion, speech, sensations, touch, hearing, feelings like fear, anxiety, grief, enthusiasm etc., natural urges, formation of foetus, the sexual act and retention.

Fire constitutes the pitta energy of the body and thus pitta is the body's fire or *agni*. When we use the word agni in Ayurveda, it pertains to everything related to digestion and assimilation. Agni in Ayurvedic terminology is a part of pitta but pitta has also some other functions.

> **Pitta** is responsible for vision, hunger, thirst, heat regulation, softness, lustre, cheerfulness, intellect and sexual vigour.

Kapha forms the solid part of the body and is responsible for the formation of new cells. Also when we are adult, our body constantly needs new cells. We need various secretions in the body. The inner lining of the digestive system and uterus is made of epithelial cells which are constantly renewed.

Kapha constitutes all the solid structure of the body and is responsible for binding different body organs together. It gives rise to firmness and heaviness to the body and is responsible for sexual potency, strength, forbearance and restraint.

Individual health and cosmic balance

Both body and cosmos are dynamic and they have the same fundamental constituents—the five elements. Just as we need the equilibrium of five elements in the cosmos for an order and harmony in the cosmic system, similarly, for good health, we need a balance of these elements, which constitute our body in the form of three energies. To imagine five elements in the body in the form of vata, pitta and kapha may sound abstract to you at this stage. It is easier to comprehend the system of three energies in the body and their equilibrium if we first understand how the five elements maintain the cosmic equilibrium and what happens when this equilibrium is disturbed.

Imagine a calm day when it is neither too hot nor too cold. The wind is blowing mildly and there is a perfect ratio of humidity in the air. Everything seems serene and calm and you feel good in this kind of atmosphere. Imagine another day with very strong winds blowing. Most of you will feel restless and unwell in this kind of weather. Strong winds sometimes uproot trees or destroy other things. If the trees fall in a river and hinder the flow of water, there is a danger of flood. First of all, the element wind was not in equilibrium. It disturbed the element earth and uprooted the trees. The trees were no more there where they should have been and they were there where they should not be. Thus, the fast winds also disturb the element space. Flood disturbs the element water as it enters into the fields and destroys the crops. Once again, the element earth is disturbed. Thus we see that when one of the elements in nature does not function properly, the whole system is disturbed. Similarly, for good health, the three vital forces or dosha of the body, made from five elements, should perform their functions in harmony with each other. If one of the energies is disturbed, you get a state of imbalance and feel unwell. If this state persists, the other energies also get disturbed, leading to ill health and disorders.

When the summer is too hot or it does not rain and there is drought, or there are accidents with the life-giving fire or there are floods or earthquakes, there is destruction. Similarly, when we do not maintain the equilibrium of the five elements in our system, there are disturbances and ill health. In other words, our system is built the same way as nature. If we go against nature, eat too much or too little or too frequently or do not sleep during the night or sleep during the day and do not care to go to the toilet on time, and so on, our system is disturbed with these anti-natural acts.

All the cosmic functions are performed with great precision. The sun rises and sets on time. Seasons come on time and the flowers and fruits appear when it is time for them. It is a perfected system that functions on its own. However, when the cosmic system is disturbed, there are catastrophes like strong winds, cyclones, earthquakes, fires, floods, Tsunami waves and droughts. Our body system functions on the same principles but it is a miniature system compared to the cosmic system. We are the guardian of this system and with our discretion and knowledge, we should act in such a way that this system works to its optimum level. If we do not take care of ourselves and lead a life that is against the system of nature, we feel unwell and fatigued and acquire a dull appearance.

Individual Variations

For understanding Ayurveda, it is important to know about the fundamental human constitution called **prakriti**, which is responsible for individual differences. This is what makes us different from one another and unlike machines, as the system of modern medicine tends to see us. Prakriti not only describes the variations in physiological features of individuals but also their personality types.

Prakriti

According to Ayurveda, each one of us is born with an individual constitution from birth. It is the basis of our physiological and psychological reactions. For maintaining good health, it is necessary to take the individual constitution into consideration.

The prakriti of an individual is due to the dominance of one or more dosha and that attributes to the individual the characteristics of that particular energy in slightly more predominance than the others. For example, the pitta prakriti individuals are sensitive to heat, sweat a lot and eat and drink in plenty. The vata prakriti ones are agile and swift in their movements. The kapha prakriti persons are slow and stable in their movements and are more tolerant than the previous two. In the mixed prakriti, the person may experience different attributes at different times and in different situations.

Seven principal types of prakriti:

1. VATA
2. PITTA
3. KAPHA
4. VATA-PITTA
5. PITTA-KAPHA
6. VATA-KAPHA
7. SAMADOSHA (all energies in equal proportions)

How to Determine your Prakriti?

You need to know the characteristics of each type of prakriti in order to understand yourself.

Table 1. Physical features and personality traits of individuals with vata prakriti

1.	Intolerant to cold and shiver easily
2.	Agile
3.	Quick and unrestricted in their movements
4.	Swift in actions
5.	Dry skin
6.	Smoky eyes and rather dull complexion
7.	Coarse hair and nails
8.	Prominent blood vessels
9.	Quick to worry, get easily fearful and in general rapid in the display of emotions
10.	Get easily irritated

Table 2. Physical features and personality traits of individuals with pitta prakriti

1. Intolerant to heat
2. Have usually hot face
3. Delicate organs
4. Tendency to have moles, freckles and pimples
5. Lustrous complexion and pinkish eyes
6. Excessive hunger and thirst
7. Tendency to have hair fall
8. Body odour
9. Intolerance and lack of endurance
10. Get easily angry specially when hungry

Table 3. Physical features and personality traits of individuals with kapha prakriti

1. Slow in activities and speech
2. Stable movements
3. Well united and strong ligaments
4. Clear eyes, face and complexion
5. Little hunger, thirst or perspiration
6. Disorderly
7. Delayed initiation
8. Slow to take decisions
9. Patient and tolerant
9. Generally satisfied

Try to find out from the above description about your fundamental constitution. Some of you may get confused to find out that you have characteristics of the two of the three energies described above. Obviously, you have mixed prakriti.

26

Mixed prakriti

You can have mixed prakriti with vata-pitta, vata-kapha and pitta-kapha. When you have mixed prakriti, different signs may appear in phases, in different situations or in different parts of the body. For example, you may be quick to react and decide, active in doing things and keeping order at times whereas at other times you may be slow, lazy and indecisive. During this latter period, you may be calm and take thoughtful decisions whereas in your active period, you may take impulsive decisions for which you may have to regret at times. Certain parts of your body may have smooth skin whereas other parts may have dry and rough skin. With all these features, you are of **vata-kapha** prakriti. Recall the elements of these two energies. You have predominance of wind and vastness of space on one side and stillness of earth and water on the other side. You have the dryness of wind and wetness of water.

If you are of **vata-pitta** prakriti, at times you feel terribly intolerant to heat and at other times you feel intolerant to cold and want heat. You may have excessive sweating in some parts of the body whereas in other parts, you may have dryness. Your requirement to eat and drink may vary from time to time. Similarly, your complexion may vary from lustrous to dull. Thus, you have features of both vata and pitta. You have the fiery element as well as wind. The wind makes the fire waver from low to high and takes away its stability. Similarly, fire produces heat and that brings the wind in movement.

If you have **pitta-kapha** prakriti, you have fire on the one hand and water on the other with completely contrasting characteristics. However, the heaviness of the earth brings stability in this contrasting state. Dynamic at times, you may postpone your work at another time. One day, you may wake up with great enthusiasm and dynamism to clear the disorder around you. Sometimes or during some phase of your life, you may eat a lot whereas at other times, have a relatively small appetite. You may be intolerant, impatient and quick to get angry at one time whereas at another time, you may surprise others with your tolerance and patience.

If you feel that you are a balanced person and your physical needs are stable, you have **samadosha** prakriti. Individuals with this prakriti are not disturbed by changing weather or climate, change of place and changing moods of others. They are mentally stable individuals.

For determining prakriti in a systematic manner, work out in three steps. Observe carefully your external appearance, then your physical reactions and then behaviour. I have summed up the process in the following table (Table 4).

Table 4. Three different aspects for learning to determine prakriti

EXTERNAL APPEARANCE	PHYSICAL REACTIONS	BEHAVIOUR
The most basic observation for determining prakriti as well as to know the state of your health is your outward appearance. Eyes, complexion, nature of the skin, quantity and quality of the hair, body structure and other features of an individual's appearance come in this category. Clear eyes and complexion and dense hair growth determines kapha prakriti. Dry appearance and a dull skin colour, smoky eyes, rough appearance of hair speaks for vata prakriti. Pinkish eyes and complexion and less hair signify pitta prakriti.	The second step to determine prakriti is to observe your physical reactions to various life situations. For example to note the physical reactions to a stress situation, shocking news, good news, exciting news, an emergency, and so on. When under stress or in a bad situation, some may have frequent stool or urination (pitta), the others may get constipation (vata), there are still others who may vomit (kapha). Some may just sleep or remain dumbfounded (kapha). On long-term stress situations like at work, various persons display diverse reactions. Some may get stomach problems or other ailments related to digestive system (pitta). There are others, who may get different kinds of aches (vata). Another type of person may start sleeping too much and also get a little depressed (kapha).	The way people walk, talk, climb up the stairs, enter into a room, answer their doorbells or telephones reveal their prakriti. Vata prakriti individuals jump up the stairs, almost jump to respond to telephone or doorbell. In between are pitta and the slower ones are kapha. Notice the behavioural aspect of their reactions. When something goes wrong, people react differently. Does a person get angry (pitta) or keep patience (kapha)? While narrating something, various persons have their own ways. Similarly, while listening to others, people react differently. The ones full of enthusiasm and clarity in narration are of pitta prakriti. Those who are too rapid and confuse the story slightly are the individuals with vata prakriti. Slow and stable narration comes from kapha prakriti individuals.

Prakriti and vikriti (state of non-health)

Your prakriti is your body's basic nature and the tendency of the nature is to be orderly and healthy. Due to external factors like weather, climate, stress, wrong nutrition and so on, prakriti may change into vikriti or imbalance, which is a state of non-health*. Nature of the body is such that it reverts back to its natural conditions on its own. But if the factors disturbing this nature are very strong and constantly oppress it, the state of vikriti prolongs. We need appropriate food, drugs and other measures to revert to prakriti. However, if the state of imbalance is left unattended for a long time, it will give rise to ailments or disorders.

It is normal to change from the state of prakriti to vikriti due to so many reasons in our day-to-day life. A normal healthy person automatically reverts back to prakriti. However, if you assist nature in her task, the process to revert back to prakriti will be rapid. Charaka, the great Ayurvedic sage from 6th Century B.C. had compared it to a fallen person after hitting a stone. The person will get up any way; however, if someone gives him/her a hand, it is helpful.

Prakriti 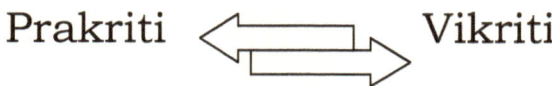 Vikriti

You can recognise the vikriti by various symptoms. As I said earlier, these are mostly 'subjective symptoms'. Always remember that you are the best judge of your body. No machine and no physician can know your body better than you yourself. Thus

---

* I have coined this word non-health to translate vikriti. Vikriti is not a state of ill health. It is a temporary diversion from the state of health.

do not ignore yourself and be always alert to the slight changes taking place in your body and state of mind.

The following table sums up the lists of symptoms you get due to vikriti in your three energies and upset your whole system. You may have one or more symptoms of vitiation. It is not essential that you have all the symptoms simultaneously. The more intensive the vikriti, the more the symptoms. But your aim should be to nip the evil in the bud, react immediately at the slightest derangement from prakriti.

Table 5. Symptoms of vikriti of the three doshas

VATA	PITTA	KAPHA
• You get up in the morning with a stiff body. • You have often constipation or hard and dark coloured stool. Urine is grey or muddy. • Your skin is too dry despite the fact you often oil it. • You have dull and ashy complexion and smoky eyes. • You get very often a dried throat and feel	• You perspire too much and have a body odour. • You get yellow to dark yellow urine and thin stool. • You get reddish eyes. • Your complexion looks reddish and you get skin eruptions or pimples. • You have abnormal hunger and thirst. Excessive	• You do not want to get up in the morning. You have a heavy feeling and wish to sleep the whole day. You feel drowsy during the day. • You get whiteness in urine, eyes and faeces. • You get whitish complexion without any glow and skin remains moist.

31

like drinking even during the night. • You have restless sleep or have trouble sleeping. • You yawn often and also suffer from hiccups. • You have fatigue that goes away after rest and sleep or hot bath. • You have intolerance and lack of endurance. • You feel often irritated and impatient.	eating does not make you fat. • You often have minor stomach related problems. • You often get pimples, herpes or blisters or tearing of the skin. • You feel excessive heat in your body. • You feel dissatisfied. • You often get bouts of anger.	• You have a sweet taste in mouth. • You get excessive salivation. • You often get a cold sensation. • You get itchy feeling in your throat. • You get nausea from time to time. • You have a sense of lassitude. • You get inertness and also depression at times.

From the above description, you will be able to find out when prakriti diverts and changes to vikriti. There are certain things in the description of vikriti that you may be already experiencing but may not necessarily think that they signify a diversion from your state of health. Some examples are hiccupping, yawning, sweet taste in mouth, undue anger and irritation, pimples or change in your complexion. Once you understand scientifically the entire system of Ayurveda, you will realise the interconnection between the nagging problems you have and the balance of the three main energies of the body. Imagine one morning, your stool is hard and dark. During the day you feel fatigued and yawn. If you catch these minor symptoms, you do something immediately; you will be fine by the next day. However, if you ignore them, the next morning you will have slightly stiff body upon getting up and despite the night's rest, you will feel tired. This state will also affect your external appearance and you may find that you have a dull appearance. You will see that if you take measures to treat vitiated vata, all the symptoms that make you feel unwell will disappear. However, if you do not take measures and let this state go on, it will spoil your internal environment of the body and you will get a dull appearance over a period of time. In the long run, you may get sleep disturbances, various aches and pains, blood related ailments, and so on. Finding that you have diverted from state of health to non-health, you need to take measures to restore health without delay.

The biological aspect of vikriti

Vata, pitta and kapha are the three energies that are responsible for all the mental and physical functions of your body. They work in coordination with each other. For example, the function of vata is distribution of energy in the body. The formation of energy is the function of pitta by digesting food. For the digestion of food, we need digestive juices. Digestive juices are produced by kapha. They are carried from one place to another by vata. Once the energy is produced by pitta, vata distributes to each and every part of the body. If the quality of the digestive juices is not good or pitta is sluggish to perform its functions or vata is too quick or too slow, the total system is disturbed. You can compare this to the postal system. You are waiting for a letter from a friend. You ask your postman everyday if there is a letter for you. He has none. A letter sent by post is a collaborative work of so many people at different destinations and the postman can give you only what he was given to deliver. For a letter to reach its destination, everybody related to this task should perform his/her function properly. Similarly, if someone has cold hands and cold feet, the error can be at the level of the quantity of energy (pitta), faulty distribution (vata) or digestive juices low in their quantity and quality (kapha).

Vikriti or the diversion from normal and natural is under or over functioning of one of the three energies, lack of coordination in the functions of the three energies or their displacement. The examples of under and over-functions of vata are low and high blood pressure. Under function of pitta is indigestion and heartburns or acidity denote displacement or over function. Excessive sleep and drowsiness is over function of kapha. Lack of secretions is an under-function of kapha.

Seven Dimensions of Being

Interrelationship of body, mind and soul

You have seen from the above description that the three energies of the body not only determine your physical appearance but also your personality traits. For example, pitta prakriti individuals tend to get angry quickly, especially before meal times or persons of kapha prakriti are rather indecisive and vata prakriti ones are rash and rather too quick to decide. Your thought process and mental state influence the three energies and similarly the imbalance of the three energies influences your thought process. With your self-control, you can diminish or enhance the anger, irritation or inertness already present in your personality. If you enhance the anger, it also influences pitta and vitiates it in due course of time. If you control your anger, you can keep pitta in equilibrium. You should think that pitta is fire energy. Angry state of mind produces more uncontrolled fire. Uncontrolled fire is always dangerous and gives negative results.

The three dimensions of the mind and the Soul

Like the three energies of the body, the mind has also three characteristic qualities or dimensions. These are:
- Rajas
- Tamas
- Sattva.

Along with the equilibrium of the three energies, it is essential to maintain equilibrium in the three dimensions of the mind. The rajas dimension of mind includes thinking, planning and taking decisions. The tamas dimension of mind hinders motion in contrast to rajas. Tamas also includes all what hinders the expansion of the mind (greed, anger, jealousy, laziness, etc.). The sattva dimension of the mind includes equilibrium, goodness, truth, compassion, stillness and peace.

Three dimensions of body (vata, pitta and kapha) and three dimensions of the mind (Sattva, rajas and tamas) mutually influence each other and the cause of all their activities is the power or energy provided by the soul. Soul is the cause of being. It is beyond sensuous perception.

Sattva—the mind balancer: Our everyday life is full of rajas and tamas. We need to work in order to earn our living (rajas). When we are exhausted from work, there is a moment of non-activity (tamas). Day is predominant with rajas whereas night is predominant with tamas. In everyday life, the negative aspects of tamas like greed, anger, jealousy, etc. are also present. Sattva helps to create a balance in mental activities and provides us stillness and peace. In Practice, sattva is to maintain stillness and peace of mind in diverse situations in life. Sattva is that inner light which enlightens our way in life, gives us peaceful and restful sleep and helps maintain equilibrium of the body and the mind.

In our modern life, there is a lack of sattva and excess of rajas and tamas. There is competition, jealousy, greed and frustration. Charaka lays a great emphasis on santosha (satisfaction) and sattva for maintaining good health. If you learn to attain a mental state of peace and satisfaction, it will not only keep you away from many modern day ailments, but also will enhance your charm. Look at yourself in the mirror when you are dissatisfied and frustrated. You acquire an unattractive look that you yourself dislike. Satisfaction is a state of mind that does not come with acquiring things or being rich. Sattvic mental state gives you a glowing look because it removes the cover of darkness from around the inner source of the cause of being—the soul and lets the pure energy radiate.

An imbalance of sattva, rajas and tamas not only influences the equilibrium of the three energies but also causes mental ailments. Thus, for maintaining good health and longevity, a six dimensional equilibrium is essential as the three dimensions at two levels mutually influence each other. Any imbalance of the three qualities of mind also influences the equilibrium of doshas and vice versa.

When one of your energies is not in balance and there are related disorders, they in turn influence your mental state. If constipation or partial evacuation persists, it can give rise to sleep disorders or a hectic mental state or nervous behaviour. Stomach problems, which are due to pitta disturbances, may enhance anger and irritation.

The six dimensions of human existence along with the soul– the driving force of our being

TAMAS

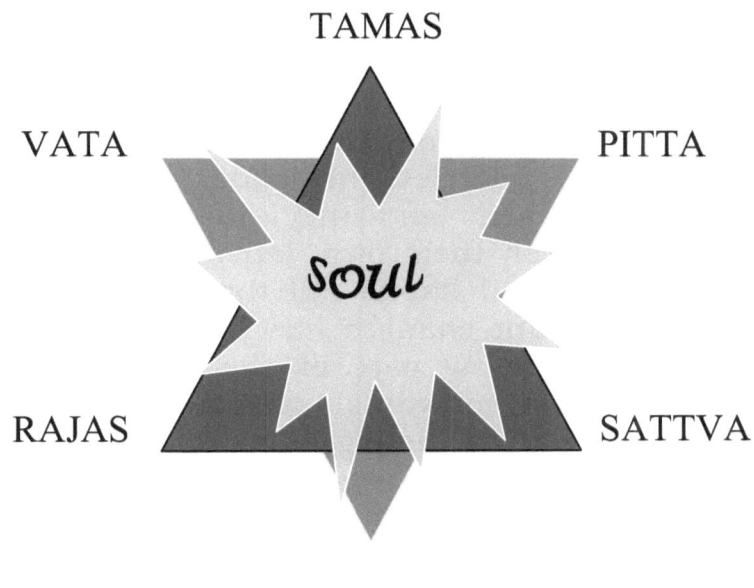

VATA

PITTA

Soul

RAJAS

SATTVA

KAPHA

One cannot think of doing everything relating to the three dosha and expect to be in perfect health. Equally important is to maintain a mental level of equilibrium with a state of stillness, calm and satisfaction. It is sattva that maintains the balance between activities (rajas) and inertness (tamas).

Principles of Uniformity in Nature

It is important to understand that the principles of the five elements apply to all that exists in the universe. The cosmos constituted of the five fundamental elements has two principal divisions according to Ayurveda: *jadda* and *chetana*. *Jadda* are all the non-livings, whereas *chetana* are those with soul and have their independent functional system. In *chetana,* the five elements take the form of three doshas or three principal energies (vata, pitta and kapha) to perform all the physical and mental functions of the body. These energies are constantly being used and we have to replenish them. After breathing, food is the principal source to replenish these energies. In jadda, there is the cosmic soul present and they do not have the individual soul or their own independent system with vata, pitta and kapha. All that jadda is, also undergoes constant changes like living beings, but these changes are a part of the bigger cosmic system. Our own individual system of body and mind is also a part of the bigger cosmic system, but that is a system within a system and these two are interrelated, interconnected and interdependent.

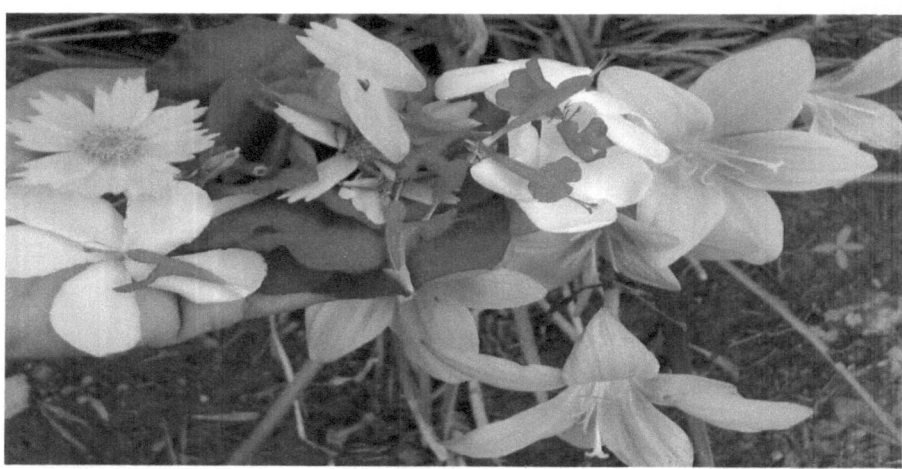

3
Lifestyle in Rhythm with the Cosmos

This chapter, as well as the following three chapters will deal with the beneficial methods of this age-old wisdom in our times. Wisdom from Ayurveda and the Vedic wisdom in general are limitless, but in this limited span of time, I am going to deal with the fundamental methods for energising the body and mind and for preventing ailments.

Living with Space and Time

Since the functioning of the whole cosmos is based upon the same principles, human beings have to coordinate their activities with the rest of the cosmos to be in tune with their surroundings. In Ayurvedic terms, it is said in a very simple way—we have to learn to live with space and time (desha and kala). Space means geographical location and time means, time of the day, time of the year, season, weather, your age and any other special circumstances at that time. Our surroundings and our activities have a constant influence on our body and mind; we have to be flexible with the changing time and space. Geographically, diverse places have different influences upon us and we have to modify our lives according to that, while taking into consideration our fundamental constitution. Let me give you some examples.

Imagine your fundamental constitution is vata. It is windy weather and you happen to live in a forest area. You have all the factors which provide you the space and air energy in plenty and that can bring your imbalance easily. You have to take care with your nutrition and lifestyle to balance the vata energy. In this particular example, the elderly person will have an added factor, as advanced age is also vata dominating. If we have knowledge of all these natural forces acting upon us and we react simultaneously, we can save ourselves from imbalance of this particular dosha.

You should be aware and quick in observing the symptoms of vikriti given in the last Chapter. Any diversion from your state of well being (prakriti) should be immediately attended to. The ideal situation will be to act beforehand and not wait until the vikriti symptoms surface. For example, if you are living in the forest and you have vata prakriti and the weather is windy, you should take all the precautions before hand to avoid vata enhancing food or any other action. With all these external factors, you should be very alert never to eat a cold meal, or eat pre-prepared meals* or expose yourself to windy cold weather or keep awake unusually late. To counteract the effect of external conditions, you should take a warm bath, have a soup for dinner and eat unctuous meals. Smearing the body with warm oil is also very helpful to neutralize the factors which cause vata imbalance.

---

* According to Ayurveda, the meals which are either bought readymade or kept in the fridge for a day or more after preparation are called *basa* and disturb vata.

Table 6. Influence of Time and Space on Human Body

DOSHA OR THE THREE ENERGIES IN DIVERSE CONDITIONS	
SEASON	**PREDOMINANT DOSHA**
Rainy and windy or simply windy	*Vata*
Warm and Dry (Summer and Autumn)	*Pitta*
Cold and wet (Winter)	*Kapha*
RELATIONSHIP OF DOSHA TO AGE	
AGE	**PREDOMINANT DOSHA**
Childhood	*Kapha*
Youth	*Pitta*
Old Age	*Vāta*
RELATIONSHIP OF DOSHA TO PLACE	
PLACE	**PREDOMINANT DOSHA**
Forest	*Vāta*
Desert	*Vāta-Pitta*
Mountains	*Vāta-Kapha*
Coastal Areas	*Kapha-Pitta*
Midlands	None
RELATIONSHIP OF DOSHA TIME OF THE DAY	
TIME OF THE DAY	**PREDOMINANT DOSHA**
Morning and Evening	*Kapha*
Midnight and Noon	*Pitta*
Afternoon and after Midnight	*Vata*

When the weather changes from cold rainy to hot and dry, the body reacts in diverse ways. There is loss of fluid and heat energy or pitta enhances in the body. If we do not take care and balance this with our diet and lifestyle, we will get an imbalance of pitta causing headaches, indigestion, skin rash, sour eyes, and so on. Pitta prakriti persons will be more affected and of course youth is an additional factor, which is a pitta phase of life. In addition to that if you take spicy food with chillies and too many sour ingredients in your food, you are likely to get pitta vikriti. On the contrary, if you live according to weather and the other climatic changes, think of drinking more on a hot day, eat some cooling fruits like sweet apples, papaya, melons, etc., you will automatically regulate your body to the external changes.

Let me also take an example of the third principal energy that drives all the functions of the body and mind along with the other two above. The dark rainy days of Western Europe are very pre-dominant in kapha energy. One needs to balance them with the addition of ginger, garlic, pepper, etc. in the food to bring sunshine inside the body. To coordinate with these weather conditions, one should eat less fatty and sweet things and should have a disciplined sleep. In addition, if you are of kapha prakriti, you should be even more cautious. If you are residing on the bank of a lake, you tend to have enhanced kapha energy. Make sure you do not restrict yourself in movement and participate in outside activities. In other words, do not give up to the weather. Since childhood is kapha predominant and if your child also has kapha prakriti, the tendency for vikriti is even more. With kapha vikriti, one becomes lazy, gets a sweet taste in the mouth, tends to sleep a lot and there may also be a tendency to get depressed.

We have not yet dealt with the time of the day. Noontime is pitta time and the inner fire of the body is high. Therefore, one has better digestive power and can digest a heavy meal. Let us say, if you are eating food which is pre-cooked or preserved, its ill effects are likely to be lesser at noontime. However, the same meal taken in the evening, when the time of the day is kapha will cause more ill effects. During this time, the digestive fire is very low. Thus, one should take meals which are light to digest—like a soup, vegetables and not a high protein and fat diet. We have lesser movements of the body after the evening meal and after sunset, the energy channels of the body gradually slow down. Therefore, for inner harmony of the body, one should avoid heavy meals at night.

Multidimensional holistic care

From the examples given above, we see that holistic health care has a cosmic view and it takes into consideration the multiple aspects of our surroundings that influence our being. This practical wisdom is easy to obtain if one proceeds with following steps:

Consider your self a part of the cosmos where you are interacting with the plant world, animal world, blowing winds, sun, sky, clouds, rain and everything that exists in your surroundings.

Obtain the knowledge of your bodily system where five elements constituting the cosmos form three principal energies and it is a system within the bigger cosmic system.

> Obtain understanding of the dynamics of the body by understanding the three energies and the constant changes taking place by their interaction that relates to our way of living and lifestyle.

> Co-relate and understand the influence of the bigger cosmic system on your smaller cosmic system.

> Apply all this wisdom in practice and obtain the ability to influence the dynamics of your body and mind.

In brief, you have to first obtain the knowledge about the individual basic factors about the holistic cosmic system where all that exists is governed by the same principles and is interconnected and interdependent. Then you have to apply this wisdom to keep your body and mind in coordination with time and space by paying attention to your lifestyle, nutrition and thinking process. Please note that the word lifestyle here does not mean the same as you are used to hearing in the West, particularly during recent years. With the Western mechanistic view of life, lifestyle is also assessed as a definitive way of leading your life. However, in Ayurveda, in this ever-changing dynamic cosmos, you have to learn to live with the changing time and conditions. In Ayurveda, it is described in different precepts—like dincharya (daily routine), saptahcharya (weekly routine), ritucharya (seasonal routine). There is no doubt that there are certain advices which are good for all of us, nevertheless, we have to act wisely according to so many ever-changing factors like prakriti, changing weather and climatic conditions, unusual circumstances like extreme fatigue or shock and so on. I will elaborate below my ideas by taking some concrete examples.

You are on a tour and you have various business meetings in different cities. That involves a lot of travelling and being at different places each day. Many times, there is a change of weather conditions as well. All this involves a lot of speaking. These are extreme conditions and they are vata-enhancing factors. In this particular situation, you have to learn to keep your balance with warm liquid meals, a hot bath or a shower each day, quietness and some solitude, and whenever possible, some breathing and concentration exercises to balance the excessive activities. Avoid eating vata-promoting or heavy foods like lentils or heavy fatty meat preparations. These precautions will help you to maintain your balance. On the contrary, if you are careless, eat cold dinners, instead of balancing the hectic with quiet, you continue to stay in loud and tiring environments (like go to a party or watch television), take vata promoting foods, etc., you will end up having vata imbalance. Above all, if you have vata prakriti, you are even more vulnerable to this imbalance.

Imbalance of one energy or vikriti, is a diversion from a state of health and will make you feel unwell, fatigued and will also lower immunity and vitality (ojas). This of course may lead to an attack of virus or bacteria and will cause an ailment.

Let us take another example. During rainy and cold days, you have to work long hours indoors in artificial light. Your work involves mostly sitting. All these circumstances are kapha promoting. You have to create a balance with hot and gingery food. Reduce sweet and fat in your nutrition. Make sure you go out for a walk after working hours and do other activities which involve physical movements and exposure to fresh air. On the contrary, if you eat fatty and heavy food after such a working day and go to bed thereafter, sleep long hours, you are likely to get kapha vikriti. This will decrease your work efficiency the following day and will lead to weariness. Kapha vikriti could also lead to mild depression.

The third example is about pitta vikriti. From cold climate at home, imagine you visit Mexico. You want to try all those foods with chillies and sour taste. You are sightseeing in the sun. All these pitta-enhancing factors may lead you to bad skin, red eyes, blisters in the mouth or acidity. On the top of it all, if you are a pitta prakriti person, you will be even more vulnerable to this vikriti. However, if you take care by drinking plenty of water, taking only small portions of sour and hot food and balance it with sweet fruits, you will be able to save yourself from this vikriti.

Vikriti and Ailments

Saving yourself from vikriti each time means investment in your health and long life. On the contrary, leaving the vikriti unattended will give rise to chronic vikriti and one is likely to undergo the following sequence:

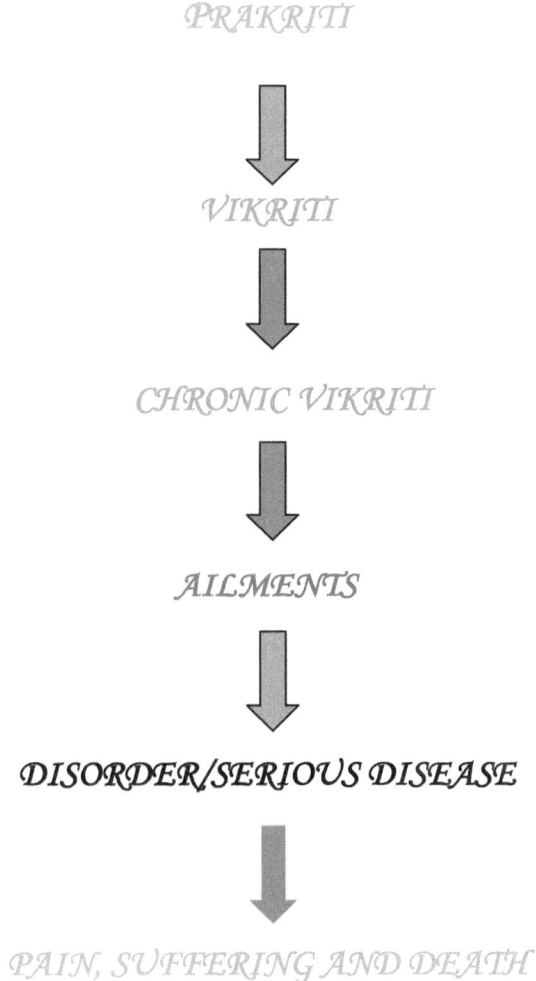

PRAKRITI

↓

VIKRITI

↓

CHRONIC VIKRITI

↓

AILMENTS

↓

DISORDER/SERIOUS DISEASE

↓

PAIN, SUFFERING AND DEATH

Balance of the three energies is constantly disturbed and reformed again. It is a natural phenomenon. Knowledge of Ayurveda teaches us to help nature. When we are not aware of the factors that bring us to vikriti, we do not avoid them to revert back to prakriti and rather enhance vikriti. Slowly the vikriti becomes chronic and in due course of time, it takes the form of an ailment. If the ailment is not properly attended to in a holistic manner, it changes to an incurable disorder that gives rise to pain and death.

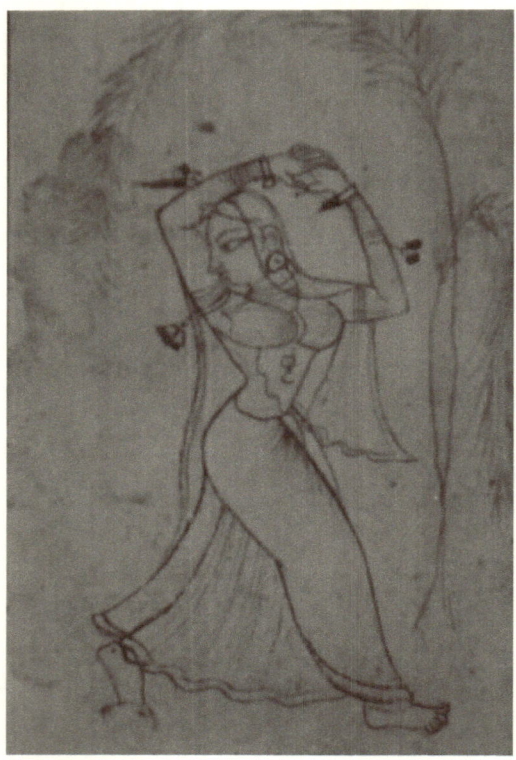

Please remember that vikriti comes to prakriti on its own, as the nature (translation of the word prakriti) is fundamentally healthy and balanced. By itself, it retrieves back from any diversion which is against the nature or is not in tune with the natural rhythm. For example, if we have pitta vikriti, the heat is taken out of the body by mild diarrhoea. In fact, one should not interfere in the natural process by trying to stop this mild diarrhoea with medication. Kapha vikriti is balanced with sticky stool or vomiting. Vata vikriti is balanced with sleep and wind release.

It is our duty or *svadharma* towards our body to help nature. diagnose vikriti and make every effort to revert to prakriti or to our natural state of being.

4
Cleanliness and Purity of Body and Mind

The accumulation of impurities in our body gradually blocks the energy channels and cause an obstruction in the flow of energy. When we do not live in rhythm with nature, the impurities are caused. When we repeatedly do so, we accumulate dirt within the body, thus resulting in many self-created disorders. Let us see how we accumulate impurities and learn to clean the body with some simple Ayurvedic methods of purification and detoxification. It is also important to avoid all that which makes the body impure. Cleanliness of the body is a constant process and the intensive purification methods should be applied periodically. It can be compared with cleaning the house. Normally we do routine cleaning of the house. Many of us clean the house thoroughly three to four times a year. We also renovate or get the house painted. Our body needs similar attention and care.

Purity of mind is equally important. As said earlier, sattva is the balancing factor for our daily activities (rajas) and the inertness generated from those activities (tamas). We need a constant check on ourselves not to divert to extreme rajas and tamas mode and maintain inner peace and harmony. Like the purification of the body, we have to purify our mind constantly by avoiding thoughts like competition, jealousy, anger, greed, etc., with a conscious effort.

Factors Causing Physical Impurities in the Body and Methods to avoid them

Nutrition according to Ayurveda is all that we take inside our body by the way of eating, licking, breathing or through the skin. In our times, we consume a large quantity of toxins. It is important to be aware of the diverse toxins in our food so that we are able to avoid their intake. Toxins accumulate in the body with time and give rise to serious disorders and ailments. It seems that even with the best of our efforts like eating organic food, avoiding exposure to chemicals and with the correct use of medication; we cannot completely avoid the intake of toxins.

The aim of this chapter is to make you aware of the toxins we take in our daily lives and how they disturb or cause slow death of the perfected system of our body. The second important factor is to learn simple methods of detoxifying the body by purification practices of Ayurveda. Intake of simple preparations taken from time to time can help you get rid of toxins and help prevent several ailments. There are some daily, weekly and half yearly practices which can help avoid ailments and disorders caused due to toxins.

Toxic Substances with our Food

Pesticides: The poison that kills insects, also destroys the life-giving nourishment on which it is sprayed and the earth, which is the giver of all and finally the water which renders fluidity to life. Each day we consume poison with our nourishment. By consuming such food over the years, we accumulate a lot of poisons and alien elements in our system. Depending upon individual constitution and fundamental health (ojas), people become victim to serious disorders in their living system, like cancer, kidney failure, blood disorders, allergies, asthma, and so on. Union Carbide Company's release of the anti-life pesticides in Bhopal accident on the 2nd of December 1984 is a good example to show the effect of these poisons on us. What happened that tragic night is happening to all of us each day and we accumulate the same intensity in our body in about thirty years as the victims had in one night in Bhopal. In other words, we are victimising ourselves to a great tragedy due to ignorance. Each time we consume the food sprayed with pesticides, we are doing *hinsa* (a violent act) to our living system and this repeated act amounts to gradual self-immolation.

Artificial fertilisers: Use of pesticides is only one aspect of poisoned food in modern times. The artificial fertilisers cause a gradual acidity in the whole system and they lead to many digestive disorders, stiffness in the body, different kinds of body aches, arthritis, falling of hair, diverse menopausal problems and inflammation in various parts of the body. They disturb the organisation of our bodily system and diminish the ojas (immunity and vitality) of the body, thereby leading to external attacks of virus, bacteria and other parasites. With artificial fertilisers, we may get one or more of the following ailments: arthritis, stomach ulcers, problems with urinogenital system, frequent attacks of external infections like virus, bacteria, etc. There could be other ailments also of which I am not aware. If you become aware at the initial stages of the symptoms and you take blood-purifying substances and adopt an Ayurvedic lifestyle[1], a normal healthy state can be restored again.

Antagonistic food products

According to Ayurveda, there are foods which should not be taken in combination with each other, as they are antagonistic to each other. Some of these combinations cause toxicity in the body and either you are sick immediately or you accumulate poison in your body which has a latent effect. It resurfaces in the form of an allergy, skin eruption or any other malady. Two most common examples are honey in any heated form and watermelon in combination with milk or cream. You will find the complete list of common antagonists in Chapter 6 on nutrition.

Intake of chemical drugs

These days there is an over-use of allopathic medicines. All the chemical drugs have tremendous amount of nasty side-effects and poison the body. Many of them have bad effects on stomach, liver or kidneys. One should take all possible preventive measures not to get sick and when sick, one should try to heal oneself with mild medicines. In case one has to take the allopathic drugs in certain circumstances, one should do the detoxification of the body immediately after that.

Purification of the Body

I describe below some simple methods of detoxifying the body daily and periodically. These methods are preventive for allergies and some other

---

[1] See my two books for details of lifestyle and nutrition: *Programming Your Life with Ayurveda* and *Ayurvedic Food Culture and recipes.*

skin ailments. One is able to prevent a long-term effect of the accumulations of toxins, which give rise to serious ailments and disorders.

Daily Detoxification with Cardamom Water

Water is life and it is the biggest purifier. The body throws out toxins through urine and sweat. We should take enough fluids so that the body automatically does this cleansing process. It is recommended in Ayurveda that our food should be fluid. However, one should not exaggerate the intake of water, like some people are doing these days by drinking two litres of water everyday. Excess or lack of water in the body is strenuous for the kidneys. The lack of water leads to accumulation of toxins in the body, whereas an excess of water is over-taxing for the kidneys. Besides that, different persons have diverse requirements of water according to their prakriti. Kapha prakriti persons need less water than vata and pitta prakriti individuals. The presence of the domination of air and fire dries up.

You should take liquid food like soups and gruels to have enough fluid in your body. A person who eats dried and salty meat products, bread and cheese (both are highly salty), requires a lot more water than a person who eats pasta or rice with vegetables, a salad and a soup. In this latter menu, there are plenty of water contents. According to Ayurvedic food culture, water and other drinks should not be taken with food, as they fill the stomach and do not leave place for the digestive juices. (see chapter six for more details).

For daily detoxification drink one to two glasses of hot cardamom water upon getting up in the morning and one glass of the same water at night before going to bed. Cardamom water is made by boiling one litre of water with 2 to 3 crushed cardamoms. Boil the water for about a minute and fill the flasks with it or else re-heat it before drinking. It is recommended to do some exercises, yoga or go for a walk after drinking the morning hot water. In any case, do not lie down after drinking the morning hot water and do not eat breakfast at least until half an hour. Morning water taken on an empty stomach takes away the impurities from your digestive tract, cleans the urinary system and ensures proper evacuation. The evening water purifies you from any dirt accumulated in the system during the day.

Monthly detoxification with Purgation and Fomentation

Purgation is recommended specially for those who have excess of heat in their body, have often pimples or other skin eruptions. It throws out excess of heat and impurities from the body. It also reactivates the functions of the liver and other digestive glands and enhances the digestive power or bodily fire called agni in Ayurveda.

Preparation for purgation: For any kind of purification in Ayurveda, the body has to be prepared so that the impurities are loosened and come out with facility.

Application of oil and fomentation: Apply some warm oil on your body and massage properly on your own or get yourself massaged. See the next chapter for oil saturating self-massage. After the oil application, do some fomentation by sitting in a hot bath with some essential oils. Use oils of rose, jasmine, sandalwood, eucalyptus or citronella. There are combinations of such oils available in the market for baths. Sit in the bath until you begin to sweat. Sweating detoxifies and makes the skin soft when done after oil application.

Come out of the bath, put on your bathrobe and get into bed to take rest. Your body will continue to sweat. Drink ginger tea, which should be pre-prepared and kept in a thermos near your bed. This will compensate for the loss of fluid from your body and help the process of fomentation. Make sure that there is no draft while you are massaging or doing fomentation.

Repeat this process twice at an interval of three days before taking a purgative.

Purgation: Purgation is done by taking a purgative substance in the evening, before going to bed. Pay attention to the following before you take a purgative.

- You should not be ill or suffering from fatigue.
- You should not be in a hectic state of mind.

Choice and dose of the purgative: In every country there are purgative plants which are generally used to cure constipation. However, you need a stronger dose (two to three times) than the one taken to cure constipation. The purgative could be from a single plant or mixture of several plants.

Sanaye (*Cassia augustifolia*) is a very good purgative for purification. Take about 1 teaspoon of the powdered leaves with warm water before going to bed.

Alternatively, the pulp of amaltas (*Cassia fistula*) can be taken. Take out the pulp from about

12-13 cm (about 5 inches) of the bean stock. Beans are between 30 cm (1 foot) to 60 cm (2 feet) long. Boil the pulp in a little water. Mash it properly and filter it through a strainer. Drink it at night before going to bed.

Reaction: Purgatives are taken in the evening before going to bed. They work inside you during the night and depending on your state of health, you may have stomach-ache or flatus before you get loose motions. The reaction time naturally varies from one individual to another. Some of you may feel a strong urge to go to the toilet during the early hours of the morning; others will need some time after getting up and have to drink something before the reaction begins. It is not important when the purging begins. What matters is that it occurs several times until there is only water coming out. If you do not purge properly and you have only one or two motions, repeat the process with a larger dose.

After purgation: Take light liquid meals like soups, rice and easily digestible vegetables like zucchini, pumpkin, carrots, turnips, etc. Eat only cooked food. Take some rest and avoid doing any strenuous physical work for the next two days.

Half-yearly Detoxification with Blood Purifiers

There are some particular plant products which purify the blood and eliminate toxin through sweat, urine and stool.

Blood-purifying substances: Certain plants are capable of detoxifying the blood and some of them are also used in our cuisine. The most common examples are curcuma, fenugreek (methi), basil (tulsi), ajwain and bitter gourd (karela). Traditionally, in India, people also use neem fruit (nimboli) as a vegetable because it is one of the important blood purifiers and not as bitter as the rest of the product from the neem tree. This fruit grows during the monsoon season and its regular intake keeps away the frequently occurring monsoon ailments like fevers (including malaria), boils or other waterborne infections.

Blood-purifying Remedies

Curcuma Milk

Curcuma or turmeric has antibiotic, anti-inflammatory, blood purifying and anti-allergic qualities. It also enhances immunity and vitality.
Dose: one to two spoons daily.
Curcuma is effective as a medicine when it is heated. The simplest way for its intake is to boil it in milk for about five minutes. Add candy sugar to taste and drink it. The second recipe is to add curcuma in a very hot ghee and add milk and sugar to it. Boil everything together. If you do not like milk, put curcuma in a spoon of hot ghee and add this to your soup.

To get rid of allergies and other impurities in the blood, curcuma should be taken regularly over a long period of time. It also improves complexion and quality of the skin.

Remedy for Blood Purification

I give below a simple and balanced recipe for making a blood purifying remedy. Some of the blood purifying substances have a dominant bitter rasa and therefore need to be balanced with other rasas.

An extremely and exclusively bitter substance will give rise to vata imbalance if taken for a long time.

Kalonji	10 gm
Cress seeds (chansoor)	10 gm
Ajwain	10 gm
Fenugreek seeds (methi)	10 gm
Cassia absus seeds (chaksu)	10 gm
Basil leaves (Tulsi)	10 gm
Neem leaves	10 gm
Liquorice (mullathi)	30 gm

Dry all ingredients and powder them with the help of a small spice grinder or a coffee grinder. Mix the powder properly and pass it through a fine strainer. If there are big pieces left on the strainer, grind them again. Pass through the strainer again and throw away the leftovers. Mix the powder well with a spoon and keep it in a tightly closed jar.

Intake: Take half a teaspoon of the above preparation daily for 15 days. Put the powder in your mouth and swallow it with water. It is bitter and may be unpleasant for some of you. You can eat something sweet afterwards to get rid of the bitter taste in your mouth. The best time to take the blood purifier is in the evening before going to bed.

If you are suffering from excessive heat or skin eruptions, too much sweating, body odour or other effects of pitta vitiation, you may continue to take the blood purifier for 30 days.

Effect of the blood purifier: The blood purifier may give you mild diarrhoea from time to time. It is a part of the purification process, so you need not worry.

Purification of the Urinary Tract (Diuresis)

This purification practice consists of taking strong diuretic products in order to flush out and clean the urinary system completely. For this practice, you need half a day free.

Diuretic substances: There are many diuretic teas or herbal mixtures that can be used for this purpose. A pinch of barley salt (java kshar) followed by an intake of liquids does the cleansing very effectively. In the West, many herbal teas are sold for this purpose. In India, a few glasses of sugarcane juice can do this purification very effectively. Fresh pineapple juice can also serve the same purpose.

Intake: Take the diuretic substance either one hour after breakfast or two hours after lunch. If you are taking barley salt, dissolve a pinch of it (about ¼ of a teaspoon) in a glass of water and drink it. Keep drinking something or the other afterwards. Take herbal tea with anise, fennel, verbena, thyme or ajwain. Do not drink ginger tea, as ginger is anti-diuretic. You may also drink sherbets or fresh lemon juice in water with a little candy sugar. In any case, for about two hours, keep drinking something every 15 minutes. You will be going to the toilet very often and the strong effect will last for about four hours and then gradually diminish.

After diuresis: The effect of diuretic substances goes away slowly. It is quite possible that for the following 24 hours you have the urge to urine more often than usual. It is essential to take fluids. Have soups or other warm and fluid things the following two days.

The diuretic substances work on the water system of our body. They are cold in nature.

Therefore, it is very important that you keep yourself warm after diuresis. Do not take rice, cold milk, bananas or other substances that are cold in their Ayurvedic nature. Take appropriate rest at least that evening. Do not take a cold shower or expose yourself to a draft after diuresis.

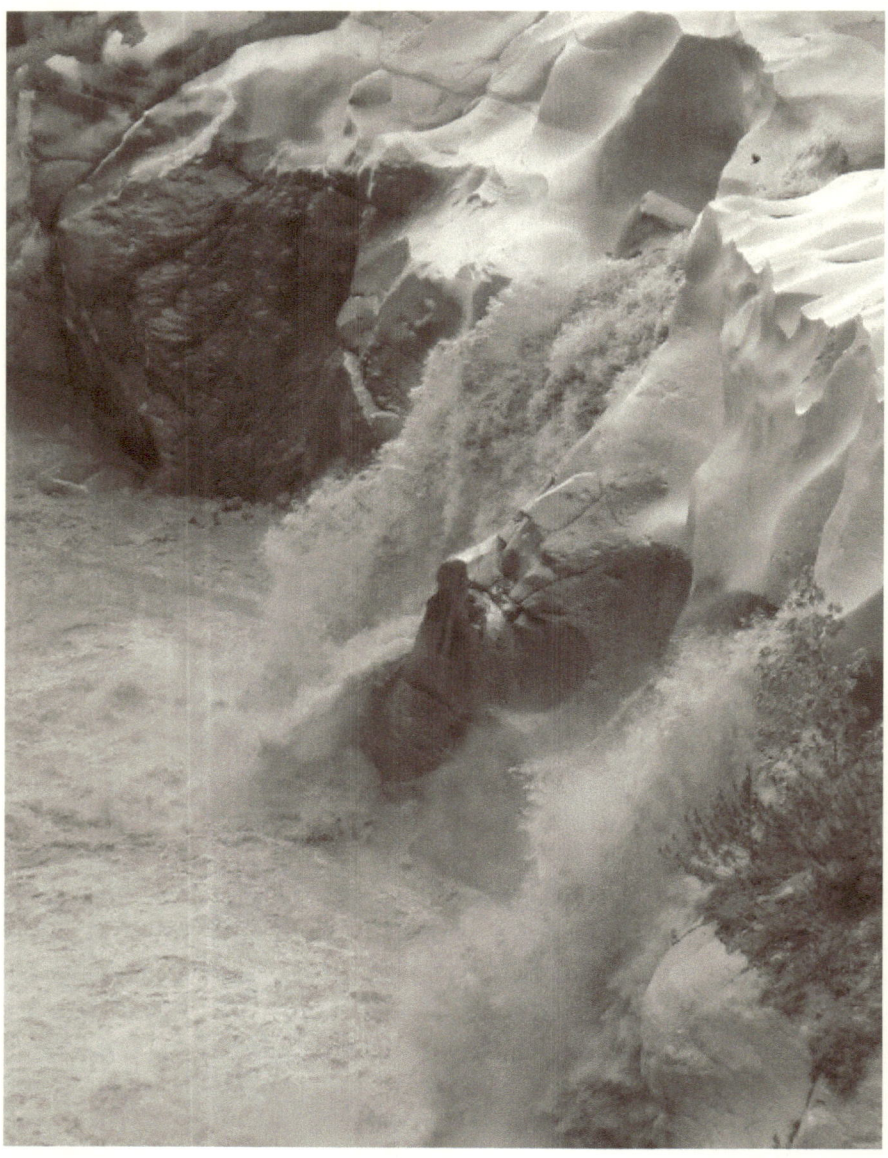

5
Lubricating the Body and the Mind

For durability and strength of the body and for enhancing resistance to shocks, external and internal oil treatments are of utmost importance. I cite below from Charaka Samhita to make you realise the importance of giving yourself total body oil treatment to the point of saturation once a week.

> **As a pitcher by moistening and an axis of a wheel with lubrication become strong and jerk resistant, so by oil application, the body becomes firm, smooth skinned, free from disturbances of vata and tolerant to physical exercise and exertion.**
> **Vayu (vata) is predominant in tactile sense organs which are located in the skin. Thus, oil application is the most beneficial for skin and should be done regularly.**
> **Those who do a regular application of oil on the body do not become much affected due to accidental injuries or strenuous work. With daily application of oil on the body, a person is endowed with pleasant touch, trimmed body parts and becomes strong charming and less affected with old age.**
> **Rubbing the body (with oil), alleviates foul smell, heaviness, drowsiness, itching, dirt, anorexia and excessive sweat'**

Charaka further describes various benefits of oil saturation on diverse parts of the body.

Head:
One who moistens his head with unctuous substances does not suffer from headache, hair fall, baldness and greying of hair. A regular application of oil on the head makes the hair firmly rooted, long and shiny and the skull is strengthened. The senses become strong; one gets sound sleep and feels happy. The face becomes cheerful and gets a pleasant glow.
Ears:
'By saturating ears with oil daily, ear diseases due to vata, stiff neck and jaws, hard of hearing and deafness do not occur.'
Feet:
By saturating feet with oil, coarseness, stiffness, roughness, fatigue and numbness of feet are alleviated. One gets delicacy, strength and firmness in feet. Clarity in vision is attained and vata is pacified. A regular oil massage on feet is preventive against sciatica, cracking of soles, and constrictions of veins and ligaments.

Lubricating the Body

You should be regular in oil treatment for attaining strength and above all for making the body shock resistant. Saturate your body with oil in the following manner once a week. After a single treatment, you will see a difference in your looks.

External Lubrication

Body massage: Use a massage mat or an old blanket for doing massage. Heat up the sesame, olive or coconut oil or ghee (clarified butter) in a bowl. You may keep the bowl in a hot water container (bain-marie) so that it stays hot for a while. The oil should be applied to the body systematically and with forceful strokes so that the skin is able to absorb it. You can do it on your own or exchange massage with family or friends.

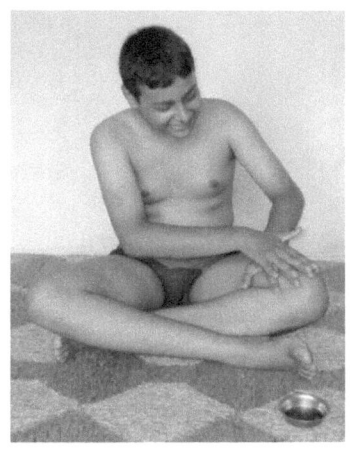

With your right hand, massage the left hand and arm and do intensive massage specially on the joints. Massage each part a number of times and keep applying oil. Apply the oil by dipping your fingers in the oil container and then smearing it on various parts of the body. Massage the right hand and arm with the left hand in a similar manner.

Massage the neck and ears and then descend to the shoulders.

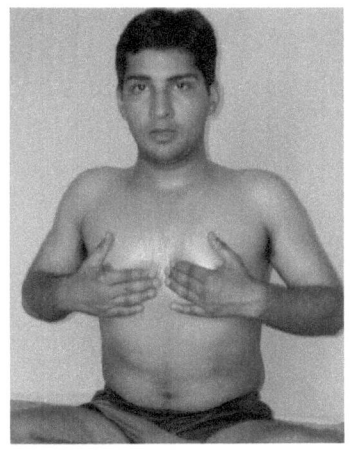

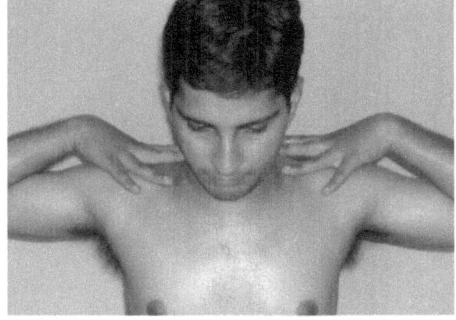

Massage the front part of the body now with both the hands by applying sufficient pressure.

Massage your face well and vigorously. Apply oil on your temples and massage them well.

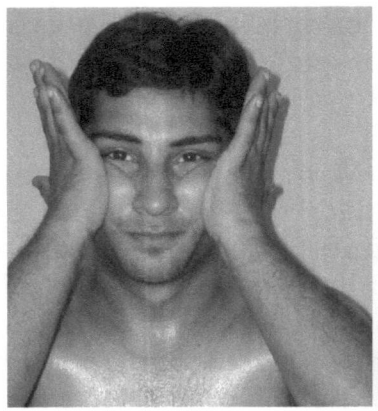 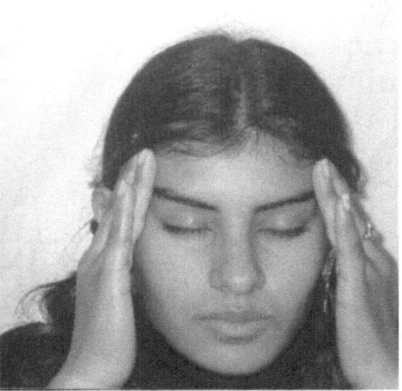

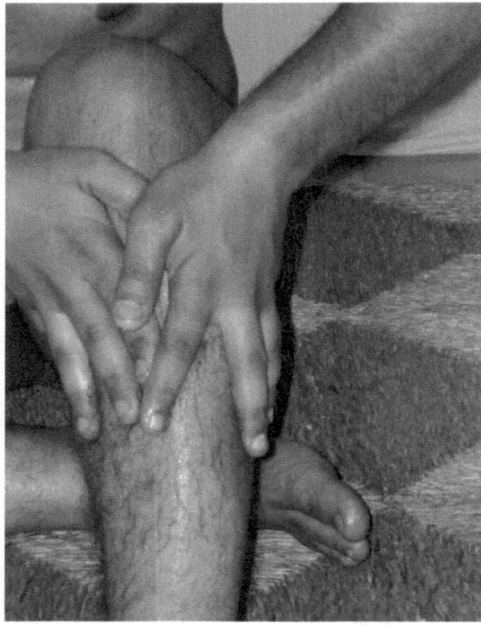

Massage your left leg from the feet to the pelvic joint and pay special attention to all the joints. Massage the right leg in the similar manner. After that, stand up and massage both your hips.

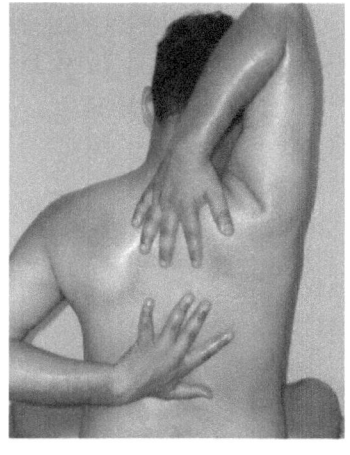

Apply oil on your back. Those of you who do not have flexible bodies may have difficulty in doing so. In any case, if you are on your own, for massaging your back well, put a piece of plastic on your massage mat and smear some oil on it. Lie down with your back on this plastic, bend your knees, put your thighs against your abdomen and hold your bent legs with your arms. Clasp both the hands together, lift your neck and rock your body backwards and forwards. Do that several times and then in the same posture rock sideways.

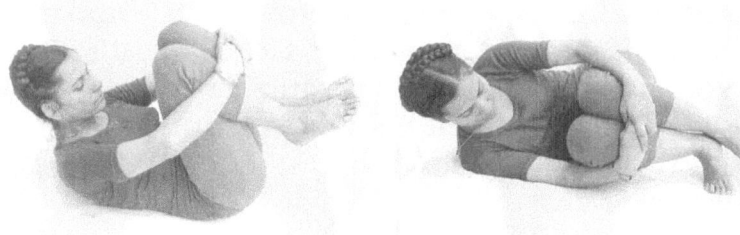

With the above steps, your body is oiled and massaged. Repeat the whole process two more times. You will require less oil and you will see that your body will gradually get saturated with oil.

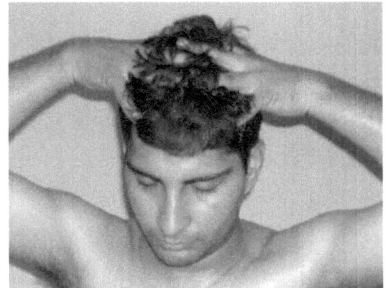

Head massage is called champi. This word has given rise to the word shampoo. On the head, the oil is applied at room temperature. Put some oil in a bowl and apply into the roots of the hairs with your fingers. Massage the scalp by moving your fingers. Once the scalp is oiled, massage it with both your hands simultaneously by moving your hands, as you would do for playing a drum.

After your body and head massage, leave the oil on yourself for several hours or overnight. Take a hand towel, wet it with hot water, squeeze it and wipe your body with it to take off the extra oil. After wiping off your body, you are able to dress up without spoiling your clothes with oil.

Application of Wet Heat

Sit in the hot bath for 15 minutes to half an hour according to your need and convenience. Do the fomentation, as has been earlier described in Chapter 4. This process will detoxify you, make your vata balanced and you will get rid of body stiffness. You will have a radiating complexion and you will gradually make yourself shock resistant.

Internal Lubrication

Like the external lubrication, the body needs also the internal lubrication from time to time. That comprises of intake of fat, usually ghee (butter fat). People with over-weight or obesity should refrain from doing this practice.

Internal lubrication is good for the alimentary tract, softens the internal parts, takes out impurities and excess fat is thrown out. The home recipe for this treatment is to take ghee in hot and sweetened milk. Use candy sugar (mishri) to sweeten the milk. Add the quantity of ghee according to your digestive capacity. You can try with three teaspoons and then increase gradually to five. People who tend to have vata imbalance should do this once a week and the others can do once a month.

Lubricating the Mind

Lubricating the mind is slightly harder than lubricating the body. Ayurveda advises us to balance the daily rajas (activities of life) and tamas (inertia and all that which hinders development of mind) with sattva (the stillness and stability of mind, with the acts of goodness, virtue and peace). The hyper-activity, emotions like greed, anger and over-indulgence should be balanced with the sattvic wisdom like the temporary nature of all that exists and making an effort not to take everything so seriously. You should get rid of the mental stiffness and see the fluid nature of our cosmos. You should make an effort to develop a sense of satisfaction with your situation and circumstances. This, however, does not mean that you should be lazy and should not make any effort. Your efforts should also be very sattvic and with detachment. Involvement and the expectation lead to dissatisfaction. According to Charaka, a mental state of dissatisfaction is the cause of numerous ailments.

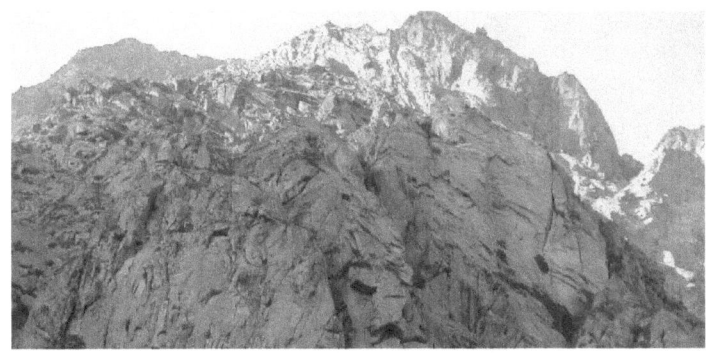

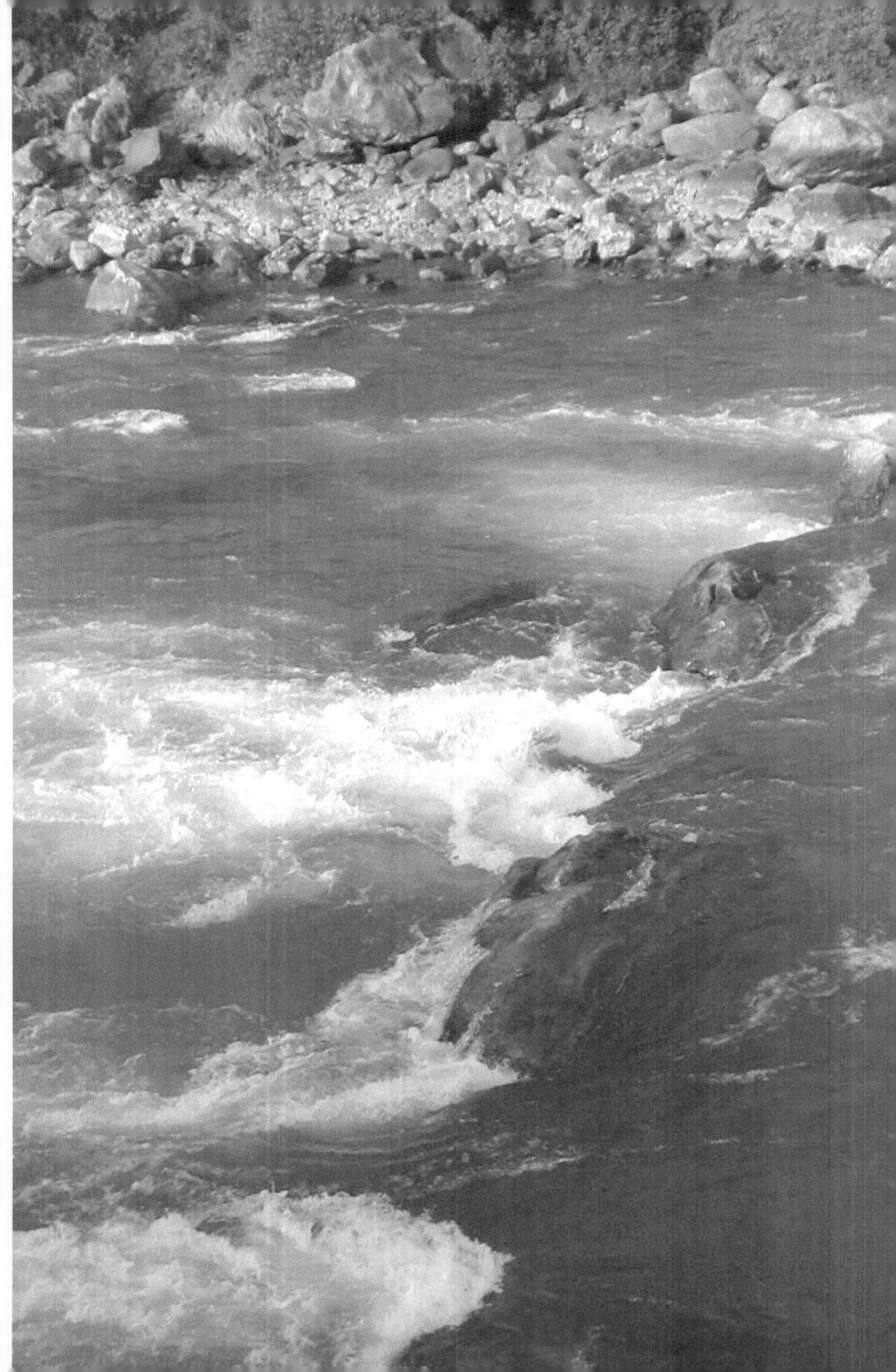

6
Nutrition according to Space and Time

Ayurvedic food culture and the modes of preparation are imbibed in Indian culture in such a way that it is difficult to separate them from tradition and rituals. However, in modern times, this cultural tradition is under threat of getting lost with the fast food tradition of the far West, which is anti-health due to the use of refined products, lack of green vegetables and use of preservatives (some of which are known to be addictive).

Ayurvedic Food-Culture

Ayurveda has very well established nutrition principles, which were written down by Charaka 2600 years ago. Based upon that wisdom, I have previously written down *The Eight Golden Principles of Ayurvedic Food Culture,* which I cite below.* By following these principles, you can heal the minor disorders related to the digestive tract, prevent several ailments and can promote your energy level.

---

* *Ayurvedic Food Culture and Recipes*, editions 2001, 2002 and 2009.

Principal Instructions of Ayurvedic Food Culture

These are the eight **GOLDEN PRINCIPLES** of Ayurvedic food culture.

1. Food should be **served** in a beautiful manner to create the congenial and aesthetic atmosphere for its consumption.
2. Never **consume** food under stressful circumstances or under any emotional restraint. If you happen to be in such a state shortly before your meal, wait for a while, do some breathing exercises, wash your face with cold water and then sit comfortably for taking your meal.
3. **Before beginning your meal**, bring your mind to your food, which is the fundamental basis of the body's energy. Look at your food and make a wish that the five elements of the food may provide you with equilibrium, vigour and good health. A little prayer or a ritual before beginning to eat helps bring mental stillness.
4. The food should be **eaten neither too slowly nor too quickly.** You should not speak with food in the mouth.
5. Ayurveda recommends **drinking** before meals or one hour after. If required to drink along with food, one may consume liquid in small quantities. Ayurveda recommends drinking only a very good quality of wine or beer in a small quantity with food. Juices and milk should not be taken with food. Water is highly recommended. Normally, the food should be fluid and should include some soup or something similar.
6. Never eat anything **before the previous meal is completely digested.** According to Ayurveda, it is poisonous for the body if one eats when the body is still in the process of digesting the

previous meal. Do not eat anything four hours after having eaten something. For your stomach, a little thing like a piece of chocolate or a fruit is also food to be worked upon and digested. Thus, strictly do not eat anything between meals.

7. Many people in the world make themselves sick by eating too much. According to Ayurveda, you should always eat as much as fills the **stomach two third and not completely full**. It means, eat to the limit when you feel comfortably satisfied and not so full that you cannot eat any more. The logic of this is that the three energies also require a place in the stomach for digesting food. If the stomach is made full to its utmost capacity, during digestion, the energies are pushed out and give rise to vitiation causing thereby various digestive troubles. This may also give rise to *amadosha*. Amadosha is the partial digestion of the food and undigested food remains in the stomach and intestines, ultimately leading to toxicity in the whole body. For the well-being of the body and for avoiding serious ailments related to digestion, it is absolutely essential to have discipline for the quantity of food you consume.

8. Never have a shower or bath immediately after eating. Wait at least two hours, preferably three hours. In any case, it is better to have shower or bath before eating. Also avoid any form of vigorous exercise after food. These actions cause vata vikriti. Going for a slow walks after dinner is highly recommended.

Nutrition is one of the four key survival elements, only next to breathing; the other two being sleep and sexuality. On the contrary, if you are eating too much, too frequently and ignoring other aspects of the above given instructions, you may be frequently ill with minor disorders, have less energy

71

level and may suffer from chronic and nagging problems of digestion. Besides that, you may suffer from *amadosha* over a period of time and thus giving rise to serious disorders like ulcers and even cancer.

To understand the essence of Ayurvedic food culture, I have made a following mantra:

Who eats what, when and where, and how and how much.

Who: Eat a balanced food to maintain your prakriti and if you have a state of vikriti, eat special food to revert back to your prakriti.

What: Eat balanced food containing all the rasas (tastes) in equilibrium but in case of vikriti, eat specific foods. Heavy, oily and fatty food will harm you, whereas light and balanced food with herbs and spices will give you health and energy.

When: You should eat according to the time of the day, year and your age. At noon, you can digest relatively heavy food, whereas at night, your food should be light and easily digestible. Alter your food according to the season. In rainy winter days, you need spicy food with ginger and pepper to evoke your inner fire. On hot summer days, you need cooling foods like sweet and watery fruits, rice and cold milk. During your youth, your digestive fire is strong and you are able to digest even the heavy food. However, during childhood, your system is still delicate and you need nourishing and well prepared food for your growth. Old age predominates in vata and you have to take care to eat unctuous and warm food in moderate quantity.

Where: At the seashore avoid excess of kapha predominant foods (sweet, fatty, cold and heavy), whereas in the mountains and forest areas, take care that you add vata balancing foods (sweet, unctuous and warm) to your menu. Midlands have a balanced climate. Desert and mountains in summer are pitta predominant; therefore eat cooling foods (fruits, salads, rice, milk, sherbets of cooling herbs).

How: If you eat your food in a tense or stressful mental state, it will do you more harm than good. If you eat your food standing or walking or you eat very fast without chewing properly, it will make vata imbalance in your body.

How much: If you over-eat (more than two third full), you will be perpetually suffering from digestion related ailments. The right quantity of food taken at the right time will provide you health and vigour.

Ayurvedic Food Preparations

All Indian food preparations are not Ayurvedic and Ayurvedic food does not have to be Indian. When I use the word Ayurvedic food, it means simply that food preparation which has balance of five elements or three energies (vata, pitta and kapha) and it not only nourishes but also enhances immunity and vitality. Ayurveda teaches us the art of preparing balanced food by adding diverse herbs and spices to make it rejuvenating.

Rasa in Food: We replenish our three vital forces through breathing and nourishment. We have six different tastes in our food– sweet, sour, salty, bitter, pungent and astringent. Our tongue indicates the taste just as our eyes see the colours. Each taste has an influence on the totality of our body as it brings two fundamental elements to us to rebuild the three doshas. This total effect of a taste is called rasa in Ayurvedic pharmacology. We should balance our daily diet by making sure that we have no rasa in excess in our food and neither have we left out any. The rasa theory is the basis of Ayurvedic pharmacology and nutrition. Each rasa is made of two elements. The balance of the rasa is automatically the balance of nutrition. The basic thing to understand is that five elements make three dosha and the same five elements make six rasas. Thus, if we put too much of one rasa, we get those two elements in excess and we obviously get a state of vikriti.

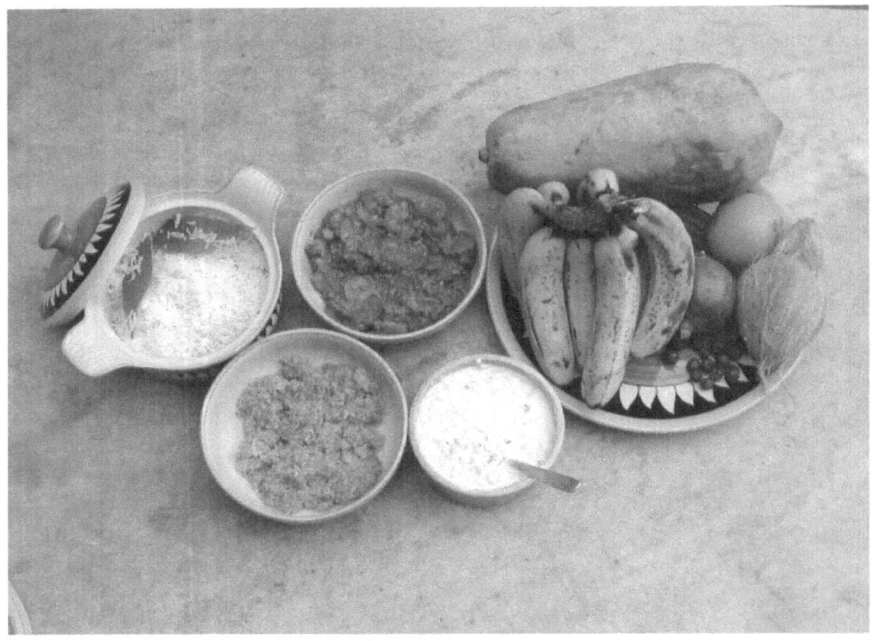

A very simple way to prepare balanced food is to make sure you have all the rasas in balance. One rasa in excess (extremely predominant sweet, sour or any other taste) will make the food imbalanced and will give you certain elements in excess. That means to have an imbalance of one of the three energies. For example, many people eat excess of sweet. Sweet has element earth and water and promotes kapha. Thus, eating sweet excessively will make you feel heavy and weary. You will feel lazy and will start to sleep too much. On the other hand, if you are unable to sleep, that means you have excess of space and air energy (vata) and you need kapha energy to bring you to sleep. A hot glass of sweetened milk will provide you that and you will be able to sleep. If you learn to understand this balancing game of Ayurveda, you are able to work for your well-being.

According to Ayurvedic wisdom, food products are not designated as good or bad, harmful or health promoting, and so on. The balance of food products is related to their fundamental nature, time, place and your requirement. In hot climate the body requires salt and you may have sodium depletion due to excessive sweat. Lack of sodium gives rise to muscular pain, particularly in the legs. You will require drinking a glass of water with some rock salt, sugar and lemon juice in it. However, eating salt in excess will do you harm, make you feel excessively thirsty and will lead to vata imbalance.

In traditional Indian households, food products are divided into three categories: hot, cold and balanced. Hot and cold foods should be balanced with each other. Balanced foods are easy to digest and should be particularly taken when one is unwell. Foods hot in nature bring predominantly pitta energy to the body. Foods cold in nature bring kapha or vata energy to body. Balanced foods provide the body with all the three energies in balance.

The Ayurvedic art of food preparation provides you the balanced way of preparing even the heavy to digest food. For example, it is said that one should avoid deep fried stuff, as they are heavy to digest. However, if one does prepare fried vegetables or breads like *puris, pakorras,* etc. then special spices like ajwain and kalonji should be added to enhance digestion.

There are combinations of certain food products and certain actions that provide immediate imbalance and toxicity in the body. These are strictly forbidden in Ayurveda and are described below.

Imbalance and toxicity with antagonistic foods or actions

I cite below from my previously published book (*Ayurveda for Inner Harmony: Nutrition, Sexual Energy and Healing*) about the antagonism in food so that you can avoid their harmful effect and toxicity.

ANTAGONISM IN FOOD

Antagonists are substances, actions, or preparations that react contrary to the nature of the body. The antagonism may be caused by the food itself, by various food combinations, processing, place, time, dose, etc. When antagonistic substances are eaten, one subjects oneself to various forms of imbalance and toxicity. Antagonistic foods produce terrible effects. Sometimes, the effect may take the form of an immediate malaise, whereas at other times a slow effect may take place. In this latter case, the antagonism may lead to a serious disease. Minor ailments due to antagonisms in food give rise to chronic ailments. Therefore, you should be selective when combining foods. Eating antagonistic food is like giving yourself a slow dose of poison.

The following list mentions some common antagonists:

1. Milk with water melon.
2. Milk with radishes.
3. Milk with sour things.
4. Honey with wine.

---

5. Honey in hot drinks.
6. Hot water after taking honey.
7. Cold after intake of ghee or other oily substance.
8. Sweet and cold food eaten by a person accustomed to pungent and hot, or vice versa.
9. Use of diet, drug, behaviour adverse to a person's practice.
10. Antagonism in processing, such as the use of food technology which may render food unsuitable.
11. Antagonism from cooking, such as cooking with bad fuel, uncooked, over-cooked, or burnt food.
12. Not eating according to seasons, such as eating nuts in summer, cold drinks in winter, etc.
13. Eating yoghurt at night.
14. Drinking something too hot or too cold.
15. Combinations of hot and cold.
16. Intake of too salty, sharp, pungent, or sour substances.
17. Not eating according to the geographic location, such as eating rough and sharp in arid zones.
18. Intake of *vāta*-vitiating substances by a person indulging in overwork, sexual intercourse, or physical exercise.
19. *Kapha*-vitiating substances by a person indulging in excessive sleep and laziness.
20. Not eating according to one's constitution.

To learn more about Ayurvedic food preparations, please refer to my book: *Ayurvedic Food Culture and Recipes* (latest edition 2009). For the detailed knowledge about the individual food products, please refer to my book *Ayurveda for Inner Harmony: Nutrition, Sexual Energy and Healing* (2007 edition). Both these books are available at www.amazon.com and Pilgrims Publishing.

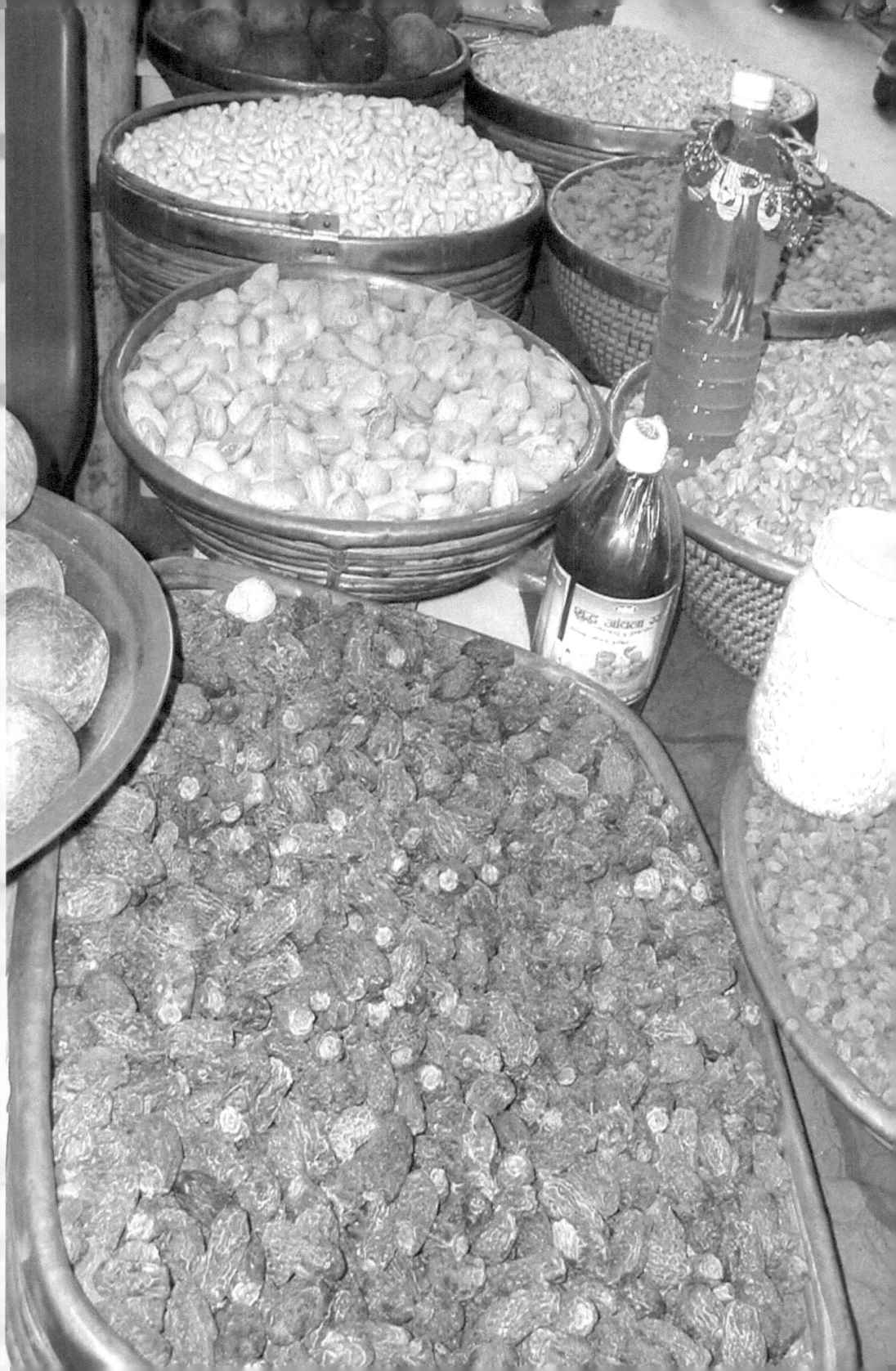

7
Empowering the Body with Rasayana

Ayurveda recommends taking health-promoting products so that our level of resistance to ailments remains high and we can enhance our vitality. Immunity and vitality together are termed as 'ojas' in Ayurveda. Enhanced ojas helps us to fight back the effect of aging, makes us resistant to ailments and give us a better quality of life and longevity. Let me sum up below the definition of a rasayana.

A rasayana is that substance or a group of substances that have several rasas in concentration. The intake of rasayanas brings equilibrium to the body and supplies vital dietary elements or rasas. It also enhances digestion and assimilation. Rasayanas rejuvenate the body by increasing ojas (immunity and vitality) and thus help fight back the effect of ageing and provide longevity.

Rasayanas are a very significant part of Ayurvedic wisdom. One of the eight branches of Ayurveda is devoted to rejuvenation and longevity and rasayanas are an extremely important part of this branch. A regular intake of rasayanas enhances ojas and gives a radiant appearance. I give you recipes of some simple rasayanas which are easy to make from ingredients available generally at food shops.

Garlic as Rasayana

Garlic has five out of six rasas. It does not have sour rasa and has the other five rasas described in Ayurveda (sweet, saline, pungent, bitter and astringent). Since garlic is very strong, it should be taken in small doses for the purpose of rasayana. Depending on a person's prakriti, it should be taken in different manners.

Vata dominated persons should take it crushed with a little ghee.

Pitta dominated persons should take crushed garlic with some candy sugar and take it with cold water.

Kapha prakriti persons should take crushed garlic with honey.

Dose: The doses of garlic as rasayana should be according to your capacity to digest. Begin with only one small clove of garlic and increase it to two cloves if you are able to digest it properly. It is better to take it regularly in small doses than irregularly and excessively.

The smell of garlic is offensive to some people and therefore to reduce it, chew cardamoms and drink plenty of water. Garlic smells from mouth, sweat and urine. Take a decoction of coriander to suppress the garlic smell. Powder the coriander and make it like herbal tea.

Garlic rasayana can also be made by preserving it in honey and persons of diverse prakriti can take it. This preparation makes garlic relatively easier to digest and milder in smell.

Ingredients:

Garlic	100 gm (4 ounces)
Honey	300 gm (3/4 lb)
Cloves (spice)	10 gm (½ ounce)

Prepare the garlic by peeling it off. Spread the garlic cloves on a flat surface and let them dry for a few hours. Take a glass jar of ½ litre (2½ cups) capacity and put garlic cloves into it. Pour the honey on the top and stir everything together with a spoon. Garlic floats in the honey and you need to push it down so that all cloves of the garlic are well smeared. Add cloves (the spice cloves, not cloves of garlic) in the jar and stir all the contents well. Close the jar well and keep it in a cupboard. Open it everyday to stir the contents or do so by shaking the jar. The garlic 'matures' in about 10 days and can then be eaten.

Dose: Begin with one clove a day along with one spice clove. You can increase the dose up to three cloves a day depending upon your digestive capacity. But always take one spice clove with the garlic cloves. Take before going to bed.

Saffron as Rasayana

Saffron is a general rasayana as well as an aphrodisiac that promotes sexual energy and vigour. It can be taken in a simple manner with milk. If you do not drink milk, dissolve it in a few spoons of hot water and then take it. For saffron recipes with milk and almonds, you may consult my book on recipes. Saffron can also be consumed in rice or in desserts.

The Latin name of the plant that gives saffron is *Crocus sativus*. What we know as saffron that is used as spice and medicine is the stamina of its flowers. Saffron looks like tiny fibrous substance with bright orange colour.

Quality of saffron: You have to be very careful to get good quality saffron without any adulteration. Saffron is grown in Kashmir and it is also imported from Spain and Southern France. It is said that for medicinal use, the Kashmiri saffron is the best.

Dose: Daily dose of saffron as rasayana is 100 mg. You can split the one gm packing into 10 doses.

A simple Rasayana preparation against fatigue

This preparation is simple and the ingredients described here are the common Ayurvedic spices.

Ingredients:

Cumin	2 tablespoons
Ajwain	1 tablespoon
Fennel	1 tablespoon
Kalonji	1 tablespoon
Dried ginger (powdered)	1 tablespoon
Small cardamom (seeds)	1 tablespoon

Grind all the ingredients after cleaning and drying them. Pass the powder through a strainer to obtain a fine powder. You can consume the powder in three different manners described below to get rid of fatigue and to revitalise yourself.

Dose: Take half a teaspoon of the powder twice a day.

Memory Promoting Rasayana

This is recommended for children, as well as for people who have to do lot of brainwork.

Ingredients:

Cashew nuts	200 gm (½ pound)
Pumpkin seeds	100 gm (¼ pound)
Almonds (peeled)	100 gm (¼ pound)
Fennel	50 gm (2 ounces)
Black pepper	25 gm (1 ounce)
Small cardamom	25 gm
Honey	1 Kg

Take a 2 kg jar and put honey in it. Add cashew nuts, pumpkin seeds and almonds. Peel off the cardamom and powder them along with pepper and fennel. Add all the spices into the jar. Stir the contents well and close the jar tightly. Let everything 'ripen' for about a week. Shake the jar from time to time so that the contents are well immersed.

Dose: Daily dose is one to two tablespoons before breakfast. You can also take any other time of the day but not before two hours after taking your meals.

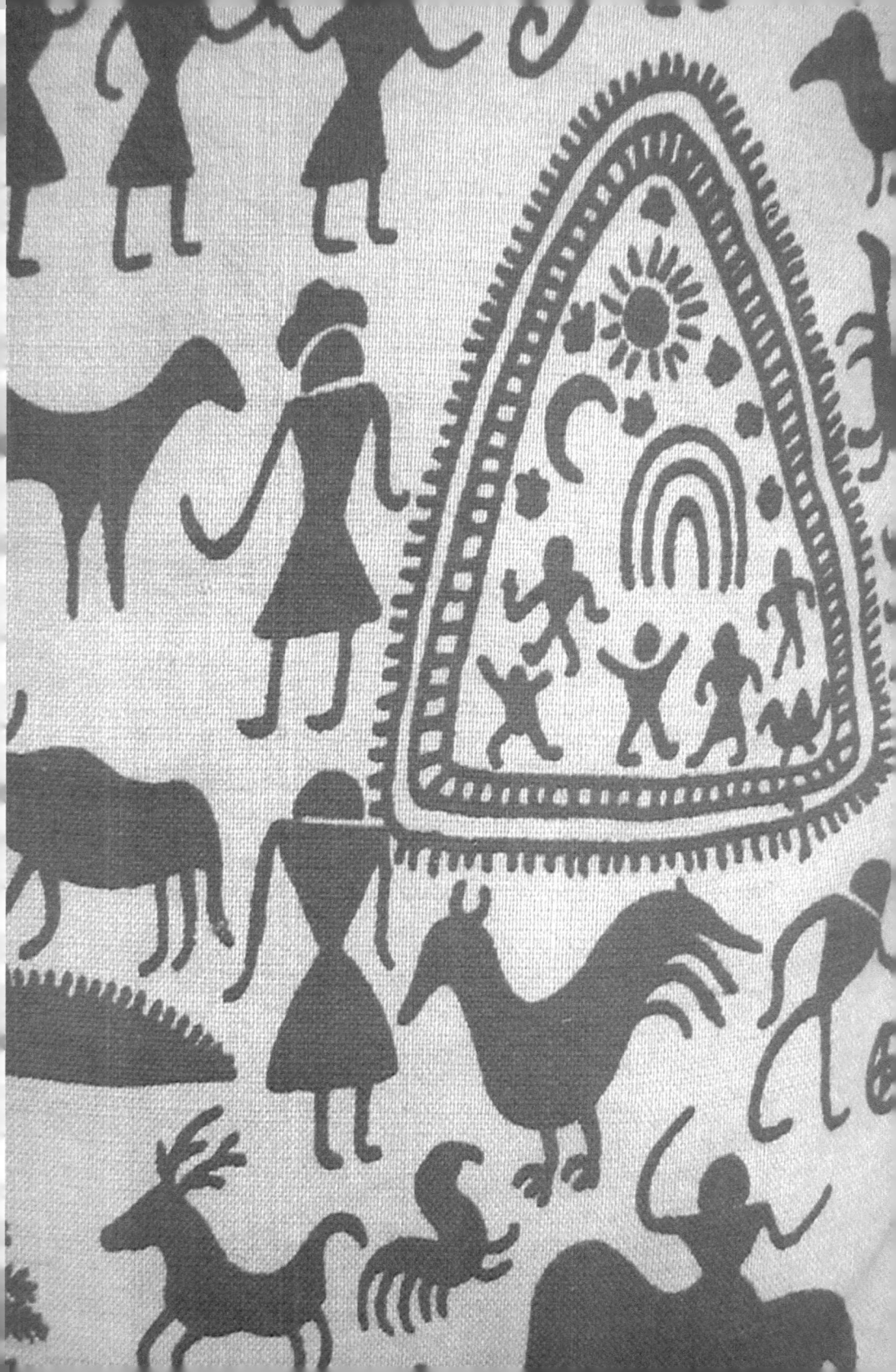

8
Importance of Ayurveda in Today's World

In this chapter, I am going to share with you some of the finest philosophical ideas of Ayurveda, which are invaluable for our times. Before that, let us ask ourselves some questions. Despite knowing the harmful and anti-health effects of certain actions, why do we do them? Why do we undertake deeds which will give us suffering? Why the national policies are anti-health and allow such harmful products like pesticides, artificial fertilizers, sweet aerated drinks, numerous preservatives and various other things alike? Twenty six centuries ago, Charaka had provided answers to all these questions. I suppose that was the prediction of the future by the sage and we are actually living in these times when we see these errors happening.

Charaka's Predictions

The sage warned us to avoid pragya apradha or the intellectual error, which is the root cause of many problems.

The root cause of the derangement of all is unrighteousness or *adharma*. That arises from misdeeds from a previous life, but the source of both is pragya aparadha (intellectual error). Unrighteousness is ... when the heads of the country, city, guild, and community having transgressed the virtuous path, deal

unrighteously with people, their officers and subordinates, and people of the city and community and traders carry this unrighteousness further. Thus, this unrighteousness makes the righteousness disappear....Consequently, when righteousness has disappeared, unrighteousness has the upper hand and the gods* have deserted the place, the seasons get affected and because of this, it does not rain on time, or at all, or there is abnormal rainfall, winds do not blow properly, the land is affected, water reservoirs are dried up; herbs give up their natural properties and acquire morbidity. Then epidemics break out due to polluted contacts and edibles.**

Pragya apradha or the intellectual error is done due to lack of dhi (knowledge), dhriti (restraint) and smriti (memory). Let me explain that in simple words what the sage meant by these three words. I take an example of over-weight, a health problem which is spreading the world over on a pandemic scale.

- I gained weight because I ate too many chocolates. I did not know they contain only fat and sugar. **This was done out of ignorance or lack of knowledge (*dhi*).**

---

* In Vedic tradition, the word "god" is used to describe various forces of nature. Charaka's description of *vāyu* (or air) will illustrate my point. "***Vāyu* is all-powerful and indestructible; it causes negation of the positive factors in creatures and brings about happiness and misery; he is death, *Yama* (the god of death), regulator, *Prajāpati* (master of the creatures), *Aditi*, *Viśvakarmā* (creator god), taking all sorts of forms, penetrating into all, executing all the systems, subtle among the things, pervasive *Visnu* (protector), *Vāyu* himself is the Lord (all powerful)."** *Charaka Samhitā*, *Sūtrasthāna*, XII, 8.

** *Charaka Samhitā*, *Vimānasthānam*, III, 20.

- I ate a lot in my holidays because the food was very good. I put on five kilos in ten days. **This is *dhriti* or lack of restraint.**
- I forgot again that I should eat dinner three hours before going to bed. Late dinners make me gain weight. **This is lack of memory or *smriti.***

For eating right food products without poisons, we require knowledge about the harmful effects of the sprays and artificial fertilisers. Knowledge is primary to any sane action and that is why sages put *dhi* in the first place. An innocent citizen, who is totally unaware of the hidden toxins in the food, consumes food to satisfy hunger and to promote health, is in fact causing herself/himself a slow death. The governing bodies are doing adharma or unrighteousness by allowing anti-health and harmful products to be sold to the public.

Please pay attention to the following in the above citation: **...when the heads of the country, city, guild, and community having transgressed the virtuous path, deal unrighteously with people...**

We are witnessing this in the news everyday in different parts of the country how the administrating bodies are playing a major role in destroying the environment and uprooting people from their homes and locations. The Himalayas are being destroyed by many hydro projects and the great rivers like the Ganga is put into tunnels. However, these projects have failed due to the porous land in the mountains and they are harming the entire areas wherever these projects are made. For the gains of a few, humanity is suffering and nature is being plundered. We have started having the effect of these hydro projects on environment and are already experiencing drought, which was unheard of in the Himalayan region.

Charaka has laid a great emphasis on environment and has predicted the conditions which occur after the environment is destroyed. When environment is destroyed, everything is gradually destroyed. Human greed at diverse levels is causing this destruction, which is evident these days from the drastic climatic changes. Charaka predicted all this 2600 years ago.

While people differ in dissimilar entities like constitution, etc., there are other common factors that cause derangements and diseases that have a similar period and symptoms and they can spread and destroy the community. These factors in communities are air, water, place, and time. Air ... not in accordance with the season, excessively moist, windy, harsh, cold, hot, rough, blocking, terrible sounding, excessively clashing, whistling, and affected with unsuitable smell, vapours, gravel, dust and smoke... Water should be known as devoid of merit when it is excessively deranged in respect [to] smell, colour, taste, and touch, is too slimy, deserted by aquatic birds, aquatic animals are reduced... Place should be considered as unwholesome when normal colour, smell, taste, and touch is too much affected...it contains excessive moisture, is troubled by reptiles, violent animals, mosquitoes, locusts, flies, rats, owls, vultures, jackals etc., has fallen, dried and damaged crops, smoky winds, birds and dogs cry there, bewilderments and painful conditions of various animals and birds; a community with abandoned and destroyed virtues like

truthfulness, modesty, conduct, behaviour and other merits, rivers constantly agitated and over-flooded, frequent occurrence of meteorites, thunder-bolts and earthquakes ...the sun, the moon and the stars with rough, coppery, reddish white and cloudy appearance. Time should be known as unwholesome if it is having signs contrary, excessive or deficient to those of the season. *

The above citation demonstrates that Ayurveda is truly a science of life and holistic. We cannot compare it to modern medicine, which largely deal with human beings as disintegrated wholes. We are made to reduce into molecules and problem in each part of our body is solved by a specialist of that particular organ. The modern medicine does not even consider body and mind as a whole, what to talk of the effect of social and cosmic environments and their effect on our day-to-day life. We live in the age of disintegration, imbalance and toxicity. Our food provides us more poison than nourishment; the air we breathe is also more or less toxic. We are forced to be pushed around to match with the hectic pace of life human beings have created for themselves. One thing leads to another and the total effect on the body-mind equation is disastrous. The gradual contamination through food and breathing leads to slow death. We continue to live but partially. The vigour and enthusiasm is no more there.

Principles of Ayurveda can help us enhance our quality of life, attain a sense of satisfaction and peace and prevent ailments. They can help us live with the consciousness of our surroundings and thus initiate us in improving our environment. They

---

* *Charaka Samhitā, Vimānasthānam*, III, 6

can also help us to form a better social interaction by enhancing understanding. Let us see some of these facts in details

Enhancing the Quality of Life and Preventing Ailments

The concept of health in Ayurveda is different than in modern medicine. Absence of illness is not considered health in Ayurveda. For example, if someone complains about a strange pain or giddiness or excessive sweating to the extent of being uncomfortable, this person is made to undergo diverse tests to find out the reason for these symptoms. If all the tests are all right, then the person is declared healthy despite the discomfort this individual is facing. Since the physicians and pathologists only depend upon objective symptoms, which are obtained by mechanical analysis of the body, the humanity continues to suffer. On the contrary, in Ayurveda, subjective symptoms are extremely important for a physician. Besides these, the outward appearance and behaviour play a significant role in diagnosis of a person. The individual is extremely important in Ayurveda as someone with feelings and sensitivity. Thus, Ayurvedic methods are patient friendly and humane as compared to modern medicine.

Ayurveda lays a great emphasis on not only to getting rid of the subjective symptoms described by the patient or subject, but to enhance the quality of life too. That means the healthy persons are supposed to enhance their vitality by taking diverse rasayanas or rejuvenating products in order to lead a better life. Optimum health means lack of fatigue and presence of vigour and vitality. Rasayanas enhance ojas (immunity and vitality) and they work as anti-aging. They help maintain sexual vigour even in the advanced years. Specific rasayanas enhance other capabilities of individuals like memory, power of individual senses, flexibility of the body, etc. A regular intake of rasayana makes you resistant to infections and thus is the greatest of preventive medicine.

Enhancing Mutual Understanding *

Ayurvedic wisdom does not classify all the humanity into one type. Individual differences are very important and we are taught to respect these differences. We are all different due to diversity in prakriti and due to the stock of our previous karma. In other words, we all have different capabilities due to our past and we should respect this diversity with tolerance and endurance. Persons with better capabilities should remain humble and the ones with lesser potentials should continue their efforts without feeling frustrated. The privileged ones should help the latter with compassion. Parents should stop comparing their children with each other and should not impose their choice of profession on them. In companionship, people should stop giving stress to each other by imposing identical capabilities on each other.

Enhancing Work Efficiency *

Rather than expecting the same from everyone at the workplace, one can organise to make best use of the inherent qualities in each individual. The selection of diverse posts can be done according to prakriti and groups can be formed at workplace by matching

---

* On the themes of Companionship and Work efficiency, I have two separate volumes. Please see the book list at the back pages of this book.

prakriti. For example, impulsive behaviour of a vata-pitta prakriti individual can be harnessed by a kapha prakriti person.

Svadharma and Environment

Our first duty is to take care of our body by keeping it clean, taking right food, doing appropriate exercise, doing all to prevent ailments and by bringing balance in our thinking process. The first duty or dharma according to Ayurveda is svadharma (dharma towards oneself). Body is the temple of the soul and how can we keep the temple dirty and badly organised?

We must make every effort to keep the body and the mind pure and in rhythm with the natural cosmic phenomena. Indiscipline and impurities lead to disturbance in the organisation of the entire system and thus, the body becomes out of tune from the cosmic orchestra. This leads to human discomfort and ultimately suffering due to ailments. When a person has disturbed natural urges like urge to stool, urine, sleep, sexuality, etc., and takes chemical drugs to regain lost organisation, the situation becomes even worse. This is the time to intervene with an Ayurvedic lifestyle and other instructions to revert to natural phenomena of the body. If we recognise the value of our duty towards our body (svadharma), we can save ourselves from numerous health hazards during our lifetime.

A person who cannot even perform his first duty towards her/his body, how can she/he take care of the environment? It is our second important dharma to take care of our surroundings and keep the cosmic five elements clean. We are made of these elements and our body is constantly replenished with these. For the sake of our survival and health, we should keep our space, air, water and earth clean and well organised.

Ayurveda: the Health-care System for the Future

The present health care systems are failing in the richest country of the world, as well as in relatively less privileged nations. In these systems, the individual is totally made to depend upon the medical community for all his/her problems related to health. Individual responsibility is missing, education in prevention of ailments by caution and lifestyle is not there at all and human beings get in the vicious circle of ailments by the use of strong drugs even to cure their minor ailments. Prevention of ailments by cleanliness, detoxification, Ayurvedic lifestyle and better nutrition are the concepts which can solve the present health crisis. It is only possible if we systematically spread the Ayurvedic wisdom through schools and colleges and through various other educational systems so that each individual realises the value of svadharma and doing something for health before one is sick. There is a saying in India, that one does not dig a well upon getting thirsty and in China they say that you do not cast weapons when there is already a war. We should always be on guard to keep harmony within our system and with our surroundings. We should make our best efforts not to let the enemy in the form of an ailment appear.

 AUM SHANTI

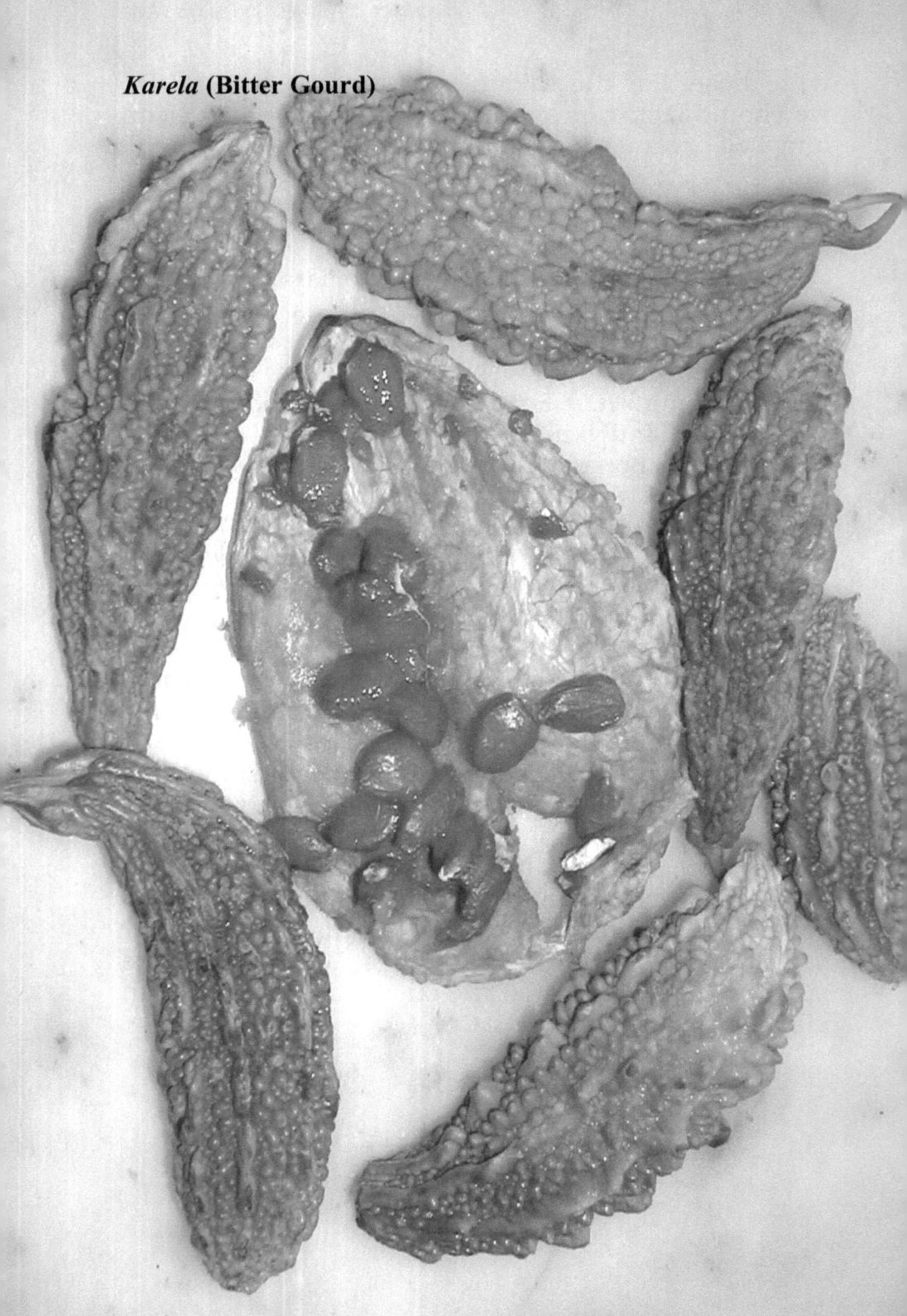

Karela (Bitter Gourd)

About the Author

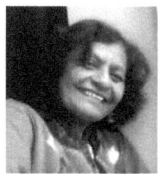 Along with a doctorate degree in reproduction biology in India, Dr. Verma studied Neurobiology in Paris University and obtained a second doctorate. She pursued advanced research at the National Institutes of Health, Bethesda (USA) and the Max-Planck Institute in Freiburg, Germany. At the peak of her career in medical research in a pharmaceutical company in Germany, she realised that the modern approach to health care is basically fragmented and non-holistic. Besides, we are directing all our efforts and resources to cure disease rather than maintaining health. In response, Dr. Verma founded The New Way Health Organisation (NOW) in 1986 to spread the message of holistic living, preventive methods for health care and to promote the use of mild medicine and various self-help therapeutic measures.

Dr. Verma grew up with a strong familial tradition of Ayurveda with a grandmother who had enormous Ayurvedic wisdom and was a gifted healer. She has studied Ayurveda in the traditional Guru-shishya style with Acharya Priya Vrat Sharma of the Benares Hindu University for 23 years.

Dr. Verma is an ardent researcher and is working hard to compile the living tradition of Ayurveda and spread it in the world through her books and other activities. She has published twenty three books on yoga, Ayurveda, Women and Companionship. The books are published in various languages of the world. Besides, she has published numerous scientific articles. Several other books are in preparation. She lectures extensively, teaches in Europe for several months a year, trains students at her two centres in India and gives radio and television programmes. A film on Ayurveda with her was made by German television in 1995 and was shown in 100 countries, in 130 languages. It was the first film on Ayurveda.

Dr. Verma has founded Charaka School of Ayurveda to train interested people with genuine Ayurvedic education so that they can further impart the knowledge of Ayurvedic way of life and save people from becoming a victim of charlatanry in Ayurveda. She is doing several research projects on medicinal plants and their combination in the form of remedies. She is the founder and chairperson of *The Ayurveda Health Organisation*, which is a charitable trust for distributing and promoting Ayurvedic remedies and yoga therapy in rural areas of India. She does regular lectures and workshops for school children in the rural and remote areas of the Himalayas to promote wisdom of traditional science and medicine. Dr. Verma gives seminars, lectures and teaches in the *Charaka School of Ayurveda* with guru-shishya tradition.

For more information and contacts for Dr. Verma's school and teaching programme see www.ayurvedavv.com and www.drvinodverma.com

Dr. Vinod Verma's Publications

1. *Patanjali's Yoga Sutra: A Scientific Exposition* (Published in English, Hindi and German).
2. *Ayurveda for Inner Harmony: Nutrition, Sexual Energy and Healing* (Published in English, German, Italian, French, Romanian and Hindi).

3. *Ayurveda a Way of Life* (Published in English, German, Italian, French, Spanish, Czech, Greek, Portuguese, Slovenian and Hindi).
4. *The Kamasutra for Women* (Published in English [America and India], German, French, Dutch, Romanian, Italian, Portuguese, Slovenian Hindi and Malayalam).
5. *Stress-free Work with Yoga and Ayurveda* (Published in German, English [America and India] and Hindi).
6. *Patanjali and Ayurvedic Yoga* (Published in English, German and Hindi).
7. *Programming Your Life with Ayurveda* (Published in German, French, English, Slovenian and Czech).
8. *Ayurvedic Food Culture and Recipes* (Published in English, German, Czech and Hindi).
9. *Yoga: A Natural Way of Being* (Published in English, German, French, Italian and Hindi).
10. *Companionship and Sexuality (Based on Ayurveda and the Hindu tradition)* (Published in English and German).
11. *Natural Glamour: The Ayurveda Beauty Book* (Published in German, Spanish and English)
12. *Losing and Maintaining Weight with Ayurveda and Yoga* (Published in English, Slovenian and German).
13. *The Timeless Wisdom of Ayurveda: A Scientific Exposition* (Published in English and German)
14. *Prakriti and Pulse: The Two Mysteries of Ayurveda* (Published in German)
15. *Good Food for Dogs: Vegetarian nourishment based on Ayurvedic wisdom* (Published in German and English)
16. *Diet for Losing Weight* (published in German and English)
17. *Aum: The Infinite Energy* (Published in German and English)
18. *Pulse Diagnose in Chinese and Ayurvedic Medicine* (co-author for TCM Dr. Florian Ploberger) (published in German)
19. *Shiva's Secrets for Health and Longevity* (published in German and English)
20. *Healing Hands: The Ayurvedic Massage workbook* (in press)
21. *Prevention of Dementia* (published in German and English)
22. *Ayurveda for Dogs* (published in German)
23. Numerology: Based on the Vedic Tradition (published in English and Slovenian)

The Charaka School of Ayurveda and Patanjali Yogadarshana Society (Himalayan Centre)

The Charka School of Ayurveda (CSA) has been founded by Dr. Vinod Verma to spread the genuine classical tradition as well as the living tradition of Ayurveda in the world for promoting healthy living and preventing ailments. Its aim is to teach people a healthy lifestyle which enhances immunity and vitality and enables them to live a life with an optimum level of energy. For minor ailments, people should be capable of using home remedies, appropriate physical and mental exercises and nutrition.

CSA aims to bring genuine and practical aspects of Ayurveda to people and save them from Americanised and Europeanised distorted versions of Ayurveda and other forms of charlatanry that do more harm than good.

To achieve this purpose, CSA organises to train students in Europe who can further spread the message of Ayurvedic lifestyle and help people with genuine massages, purification practices, nutrition and other practical aspects of Ayurveda. The school is in association with the most learned persons of Ayurveda in India and several exclusive persons involved in health education in Europe.

The object of Patanjali Yogadarshana Society is to spread the message of Patanjali in the world. The wisdom of the Yoga Sutras is not only beneficial for the yogis but also for our day-to-day normal life. Its aim is to enhance *sattva* or the inner stillness and peace in the world as well as in the individual minds. With years of research on Yoga and Ayurveda, Dr. Verma has founded the Ayurvedic Yoga and has written a book on the subject.

Himalayan Centre

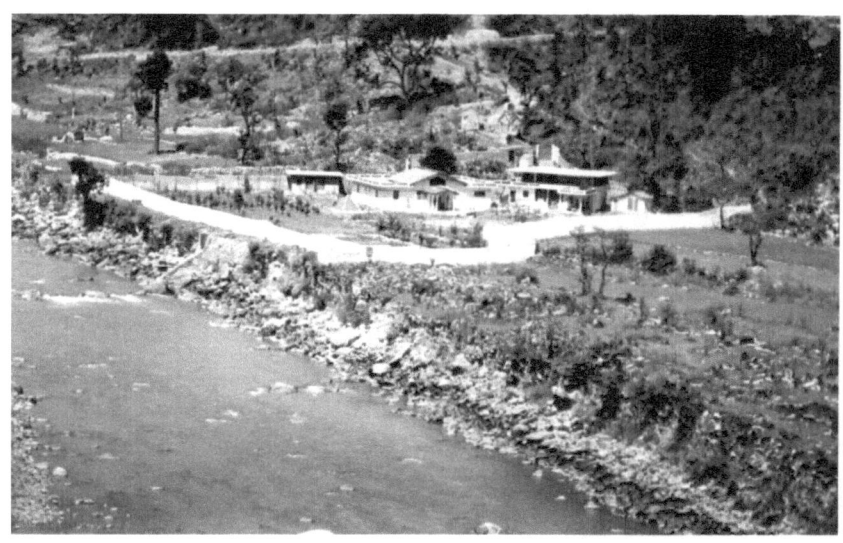

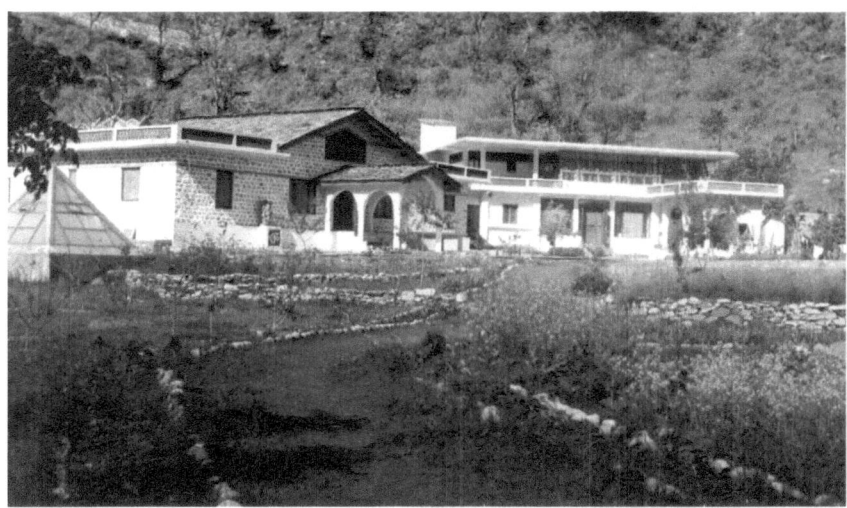

Lectures, Seminars and Training Programmes for Charaka School of Ayurveda

To get detailed information on the Charaka School of Ayurveda, as well as our other programmes in India and Europe, visit our website or e-mail to the following address:

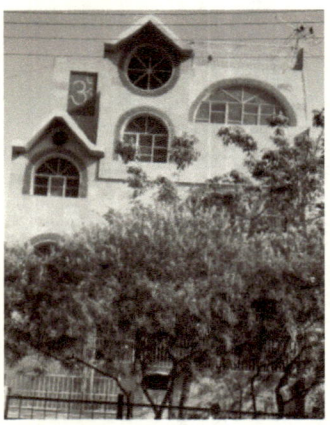

**The Ayurveda Health Organisation
A-130, Sector 26, Noida 201301,
U.P., India**
Tel. 0091 (0)120 2527820 or (0)
9873704205 or (0)9412224820
www.ayurvedavv.com
ayurvedavv@yahoo.com
ayurvedavv@gmail.com

www.ingramcontent.com/pod-product-compliance
Lightning Source LLC
Chambersburg PA
CBHW050414290526
45786CB00003B/1260